Theories of Uncertainty and Risk across Different Modernities

Setting out to challenge various common assumptions in risk research, this collection explores how uncertainty is handled in a range of social contexts across the globe. Social science research often emphasises the salience of risk and uncertainty for grasping the dynamics of late-modern societies, with theoretical frameworks tending to associate the emergence of risk with particular, fairly homogenous, European or 'North-Western' paths of modernisation. These theoretical narratives can be seen as shaping various assumptions regarding 'risk cultures', not least associations with post-traditional, largely secular and liberal characteristics. Risk is therefore analysed in terms of modern, active, 'rational' citizens, meanwhile faith, hope or magic are implicitly relegated to the past, the oriental, the passive and/or the irrational.

Central to the book is the consideration of risk across a range of different modernities. While the precise meaning and organisational processes of risk vary, we see the common combining of risk, faith, magic and hope as people go forward amid uncertain circumstances. Whether seeking health amid illness, survival amid flooding, or safety amid migration, we explore the pertinence of risk around the globe. We also stress the ubiquity of faith and the magical in various modern settings.

This book was originally published as a special issue of *Health, Risk & Society*.

Patrick Brown is Associate Professor in the Department of Sociology at the University of Amsterdam, The Netherlands. He is Deputy Editor of *Health, Risk & Society* and has published widely on topics of trust, hope, risk and related ways in which organisations, groups and individuals handle uncertainty.

Theories of Uncertainty and Risk across Different Modernities

Edited by
Patrick Brown

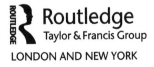

LONDON AND NEW YORK

First published 2018 by Routledge

2 Park Square, Milton Park, Abingdon, Oxfordshire OX14 4RN
52 Vanderbilt Avenue, New York, NY 10017

Routledge is an imprint of the Taylor & Francis Group, an informa business

First issued in paperback 2019

British Library Cataloguing in Publication Data
A catalogue record for this book is available from the British Library

ISBN 13: 978-1-138-08058-4 (hbk)
ISBN 13: 978-0-367-26472-7 (pbk)

Typeset in Times New Roman
by RefineCatch Limited, Bungay, Suffolk

Publisher's Note
The publisher accepts responsibility for any inconsistencies that may have
arisen during the conversion of this book from journal articles to book chapters,
namely the possible inclusion of journal terminology.

Disclaimer
Every effort has been made to contact copyright holders for their permission to
reprint material in this book. The publishers would be grateful to hear from any
copyright holder who is not here acknowledged and will undertake to rectify
any errors or omissions in future editions of this book.

Contents

Citation Information   vii
Notes on Contributors   ix
Acknowledgements   xi

1. Theorising uncertainty and risk across different modernities: considering
   insights from 'non-North-Western' studies   1
   Patrick Brown

2. Engaging with risk in non-Western settings: an editorial   12
   Nicola Desmond

3. Anthropology and risk: insights into uncertainty, danger and blame from
   other cultures: a review essay   21
   Andy Alaszewski

4. Faith and uncertainty: migrants' journeys between Indonesia, Malaysia
   and Singapore   42
   Loïs Bastide

5. Applying the risk society thesis within the context of flood risk and
   poverty in Jakarta, Indonesia   62
   Roanne van Voorst

6. Coping with health-related uncertainties and risks in Rakhine (Myanmar)   79
   Celine Coderey

7. Performing prevention: risk, responsibility, and reorganising the future
   in Japan during the H1N1 pandemic   101
   Mari J. Armstrong-Hough

8. Purity and danger: shamans, diviners and the control of danger in
   premodern Japan as evidenced by the healing rites of the Aogashima
   islanders   118
   Jane Alaszewska and Andy Alaszewski

Index   143

Citation Information

The chapters in this book were originally published in *Health, Risk & Society*, volume 17, issue 3–4 (April–June 2015). When citing this material, please use the original page numbering for each article, as follows:

Chapter 1
Theorising uncertainty and risk across different modernities: considering insights from 'non-North-Western' studies
Patrick Brown
Health, Risk & Society, volume 17, issue 3–4 (April–June 2015), pp. 185–195

Chapter 2
Engaging with risk in non-Western settings: an editorial
Nicola Desmond
Health, Risk & Society, volume 17, issue 3–4 (April–June 2015), pp. 196–204

Chapter 3
Anthropology and risk: insights into uncertainty, danger and blame from other cultures – A review essay
Andy Alaszewski
Health, Risk & Society, volume 17, issue 3–4 (April–June 2015), pp. 205–225

Chapter 4
Faith and uncertainty: migrants' journeys between Indonesia, Malaysia and Singapore
Loïs Bastide
Health, Risk & Society, volume 17, issue 3–4 (April–June 2015), pp. 226–245

Chapter 5
Applying the risk society thesis within the context of flood risk and poverty in Jakarta, Indonesia
Roanne van Voorst
Health, Risk & Society, volume 17, issue 3–4 (April–June 2015), pp. 246–262

Chapter 6
Coping with health-related uncertainties and risks in Rakhine (Myanmar)
Celine Coderey
Health, Risk & Society, volume 17, issue 3–4 (April–June 2015), pp. 263–284

Chapter 7

Performing prevention: risk, responsibility, and reorganising the future in Japan during the H1N1 pandemic
Mari J. Armstrong-Hough
Health, Risk & Society, volume 17, issue 3–4 (April–June 2015), pp. 285–301

Chapter 8

Purity and danger: shamans, diviners and the control of danger in premodern Japan as evidenced by the healing rites of the Aogashima islanders
Jane Alaszewska and Andy Alaszewski
Health, Risk & Society, volume 17, issue 3–4 (April–June 2015), pp. 302–325

For any permission-related enquiries please visit:
http://www.tandfonline.com/page/help/permissions

Notes on Contributors

Jane Alaszewska is based at the School of Oriental and African Studies, University of London, London, UK.

Andy Alaszewski is Emeritus Professor of Health Studies at the Centre for Health Services Studies, University of Kent, Canterbury, UK.

Mari J. Armstrong-Hough is Associate Research Scientist in Epidemiology at the School of Public Health, Yale University, New Haven, USA.

Loïs Bastide is a Faculty Member at the Department of Sociology, University of Geneva, Switzerland.

Patrick Brown is Associate Professor at the Department of Sociology, the University of Amsterdam, The Netherlands.

Celine Coderey is a Research Fellow at the Asia Research Institute, STS Cluster, National University of Singapore.

Nicola Desmond heads the Malawi-Liverpool-Wellcome Trust Clinical Research Programme in Malawi and is a Senior Lecturer at the Liverpool School of Tropical Medicine, Liverpool, UK.

Roanne van Voorst is a Postdoctoral Researcher at the International Institute of Social Studies (ISS), Erasmus University Rotterdam, The Netherlands.

Acknowledgements

As editor of this volume, and on behalf of the other authors, I express a great deal of gratitude to Andy Alaszewski whose input was vital to this collection. It was Andy who founded the journal and moreover the annual theory-focused special issues of which this edited volume forms a part. Alongside two valuable articles in this collection, Andy also devoted a lot of time and energy when providing very thorough comments on various manuscripts, especially regarding structure and prose. The collection as a whole is a lot stronger as a result of this.

Patrick Brown, Amsterdam, 2015.

Theorising uncertainty and risk across different modernities: considering insights from 'non-North-Western' studies

Patrick Brown

In this editorial I introduce a range of articles which constitute the second annual special issue of this journal focusing on social theories of risk and uncertainty. I explain and explore the underlying logic and theoretical location of the issue in terms of various tensions within the common association of risk with a very specific process of post-Enlightenment modernisation. I then explore a number of these concerns further in relation to and by way of introducing the guest editorial, a review article and five original research articles of the special issue. A few of the most pertinent and recurring themes across these articles – such as the combining of rational-technical approaches to uncertainty with traditional-magical ones, the salience of faith-based approaches and their agentic qualities, and the logic by which different strategies are combined, 'bricolaged' or syncretised – are denoted as especially salient for researching risk and uncertainty within northern European contexts, where the roles of faith, tradition and magic in dealing with uncertainty remain neglected topics. I conclude by linking these reflections to an introduction of the central topics for the 2016 theory special issue and point potential authors towards our call for papers.

Introduction: locating risk within one distinct reflexive modernisation process?

The origins of this 2015 special issue on social theories of risk and uncertainty can be found in the last issue of this journal published in 2014. The insightful study of Mieulet and Claeys (2014) into public health risk policies, their implementation and reception within Martinique and French Guyana raised a whole host of interesting theoretical and conceptual conundrums – especially when an earlier version of this paper was presented at the 2013 European Sociological Association conference in Torino. That these overseas departments are legally and organisationally speaking part of the French state and the European Union, yet characterised by quite distinct (post-colonial) historico-cultural structures, indicates various interesting analytical questions regarding practices of risk, governmentality and resistance within contrasting (non-)Western contexts (compare with Foucault, 1974/1994).

That these two components of France lie several thousand miles west of the French mainland underlines an awkwardness in employing a 'non-Western' epithet for denoting societal contexts which might better be described as developing through alternative or different modernities (see also Desmond, 2015). Foucauldian thought has been highly influential within critical sociologies and anthropologies of risk, especially in relation to public health, and has guided an emphasis upon the salience of a rather specific trajectory of scientific knowledge and statecraft transformation, as has emerged within north-western Europe. More recent tendencies within these evolving configurations of welfare state apparatus and their related subjectivities have been characterised in terms of risk. Whereas Foucault himself denoted important nuances and variations in the timing of developments across France, Germany and Britain (for example, Foucault, 1974/1994, p. 137), connotations of a more or less common north-west-European development in knowledge formats, institutions and the various ways by which these 'make' modern subjects would seem to underlie many recent studies offering critical governmentality accounts of risk.

Although Beck's work (for example, 1992) on reflexive modernisation is a rather different breed of theoretical project, his thesis also suggests a quite specific historical trajectory. Beck was importantly influenced by Habermasian thinking (van Loon, 2013), which in turn involves a particular Frankfurt School orientation towards tensions in Marxist theory of advanced capitalist societal development (Outhwaite, 2009) and the legitimation problems which appear within a very specific set of circumstances faced by a small number of late-modern welfare states at a particular moment in their development (Habermas, 1976). This intellectual background, as well as the more current circumstances which featured within Beck's (1992) earlier analyses, led him similarly towards a distinctively northern European and (at times) decidedly German-centric analysis of risk politics (see van Voorst, 2015).

Many of these analytical concerns can be traced further back to Weberian understandings of modern societies, the dysfunctional propensities of their organisations and various related problems which continued to define a number of the main debates of sociological theory in the later twentieth century. At the heart of these was the attempt to explain the development of a peculiar format of 'rationalism' (Brubaker, 1984, p. 8) which came to characterise those societies which can be loosely bracketed as modern, 'Western' and advanced capitalist. This same rationalisation process has often been considered essential to the proliferation of risk as a way of handling uncertain futures, as well as making sense of that which has already gone wrong (Alaszewski & Burgess, 2007; Rothstein, 2006), which for some has been primarily bound up with processes of 'disenchantment' in the face of suffering (Wilkinson, 2010).

More or less implicit within these theoretical traditions for analysing risk, its institutional and identity-related challenges (Beck, 1992; Giddens, 1991; Rothstein, 2006; Wilkinson, 2010) are assumptions which locate risk within a certain type of post-industrial society seen as possessing a combination of post-traditional, largely secular and liberal characteristics – where these have regularly come to be viewed as intrinsic to risk. For while Douglas (for example, 1992) has drawn attention to varying concerns with differing 'risks' across many contrasting forms of societal formation, it is often implied that living with 'dangers' or misfortune in central Africa, for example, entails a quite different set of subjectivities than those generated through living with 'risks' in northern Europe (see Desmond, 2015 for a more nuanced view) – primarily because of different cosmologies, civil society formations and political relationships between subjects and states.

In these senses more critical studies of risk have usually been focused upon social contexts in the global north which are assumed to be distinguished through their predominantly secular world views. After all, where more positive or problematic futures are understood by social actors as resting 'in God's hands', or as a function of 'God's will', then risk – and the qualities of control, agency and scientific knowledge with which it is connected – might be seen as less relevant and 'accidents' (and the many uncertainties these give rise to) would be impossible (Green in Heyman & Brown, 2013). The emergence of an increasing contestation of notions of divine providence through, for example, Spinoza's conceptualisation of the *remoteness* of God from the causality of things (Watt, 1972, p. 174), is typically seen as unique to and defining of a European Enlightenment path in at least two fundamental ways:

First, the dissemination of such understandings and a related growing disenchantment with religious cosmologies are often implied to be fairly complete within northern Europe, less fundamental in the case of the (southern) United States, for example, and much more partial or non-existent across the global south. Theories of risk as a product of post-Enlightenment development would, on the one hand, seem to suggest that risk-related rationalities and reflexivity would only be found in the most 'modern' of contexts (in a very narrow sense), yet, on the other hand, associate risk with globalising processes of mediatised social change across a much broader array of global contexts (see Mythen, 2007, p. 793; van Voorst, 2015).

Second, the work of Spinoza, alongside later Enlightenment scholars, emphasised the salience of doubt and the contestation of traditional fundaments of knowledge to the extent that an intensification of uncertainty was held to be defining of what it was to live in modernity. A similar claim has been made by various influential sociologists (for example, Beck, 1992; Giddens, 1991) when placing the problem of uncertainty at the heart of late-modern lived experiences, following what could be described as a reflexivity or disenchantment towards science and various modern-progressive narratives (Wilkinson, 2010). Yet these understandings of the unusual and distinctive qualities of uncertainty and doubt faced by (late-)moderns typically make little effort to compare these lived experiences with those of other actors in other social settings across space and time. When such a comparison is made, manifold and intense experiences of uncertainty seem to be far more common across a diverse range of social settings. That is not to say that exactly the same types of uncertainties and doubts are grappled with. But acute and enduring forms of living amidst uncertainty are in no way limited to northern European (late-)modernity (see for example Coderey, 2015).

Drawing on the collection of original research articles, a review article and a guest editorial which make up this special issue, I will consider some of these tensions and problematise some of the assumptions linking risk to one particular modernity. In the next section, through an overview of the contents of the issue, I emphasise the enduring presence and combining of more rational-technical approaches to future dangers within more traditional societies and different modernities. In the latter section and conclusion I then move to reflect on the continuing presence of religious and magical approaches to uncertainty within northern European societal contexts and how the analytical frameworks presented in this issue may be highly instructive to analyses of risk as a tool of handling uncertainty within northern European settings. Following on from this, and echoing some of the analyses brought together in this issue, I will then introduce a consideration of the syncretic or 'bricolaging' (Horlick-Jones, Walls, & Kitzinger, 2007) approaches to uncertainty which will form a central focus of investigation within the next theory special issue to be published in 2016.

Themes arising within the special issue: multiple rationalities across many different modernities

As Alaszewski (2015) emphasises within his review article in this issue, crude Whig-historical narratives assuming a progressive shift from approaches to danger based on magic to approaches based on the systematic refinement of knowledge and its technical application ('rationality' in its narrow sense) became increasingly untenable following Malinowski's (1999) classic study of Trobriand Islanders who had long combined both magic *and* technical rationality when managing risks related to long sea journeys. Important to this review of a number of classic anthropological studies, focusing on their analyses of approaches to uncertainty, is a paradigmatic shift in the late nineteenth and early twentieth century away from a standpoint of cultural superiority towards one of greater respect and attempts to learn from other cultures. This turn later facilitated the comparison of cultures of risk across societal contexts (Douglas, 1992; Douglas & Wildavsky, 1983) although, as Alaszewski (2015) observes, Douglas remains an under-used theoretical basis of empirical exploration. The related dearth of historical-comparative studies which explore the evolving nature of different modernisation processes and the power dynamics through which these are driven leads to an impoverished grasp of risk and its cultural underpinnings.

Desmond's (2015) guest editorial, informed by fieldwork experiences in sub-Saharan African contexts over a number of years, provides much food for thought on this latter topic, considering as she does the complex ways in which etic social-scientific notions of 'risk' are more or less closely reflected within local practices and emic (Swahili) terms regarding experiences of uncertainty. In many sub-Saharan contexts, ostensibly traditional and magical understandings and practices, such as sorcery or witchcraft, have not so much been replaced by colonial and post-colonial processes of 'development' as reworked and 'reinvented' within such contexts. Part of the enduring demand for witch-doctor practices is seemingly related to the uncertainty created amidst the social, cultural and economic upheavals brought about by development pressures and the continuing need to make 'meaning' amidst experiences of social change (Desmond, 2015). The analysis developed within Desmond's editorial draws special attention to interwovenness of conceptions of *misfortune* in relation to the past and conceptions of *risk* in relation to the future, as reflected in emic accounts. These hybrid understandings emerge within cultural contexts of risk which are 'situated between the two worlds of tradition and modernity' (Desmond, 2015, pp. 196–204). Desmond's arguments, drawing on African studies literatures to emphasise 'continuity' rather than a break with the past, have important implications for the study of risk in sub-Saharan Africa but furthermore in northern European and North American contexts where the enduring nature of the traditional and magical, as apparent within language, practices and cultural frames, has tended to be overlooked (Bastide, 2015).

Following this line of exploration, Japan represents a fascinating example of an advanced capitalist society in the global north where, at least to a European gaze, the enduring legacy of traditional culture is more palpably co-present *alongside* the late-modern. Once again the interwovenness of the traditional and modern is made visible within the analysis developed by Armstrong-Hough (2015) when considering various accounts of 'gargling' in response to the risk posed by the H1N1 virus pandemic. On the one hand gargling resonates with a long tradition of health-seeking approaches in Japanese culture which may be understood in relation to a particularly characteristic Japanese cultural concern with boundary spaces between the inside and outside

(Ohnuki-Tierney, 1984). Yet on the other hand doctors are aware that the evidence-base for gargling from studies carried out in Japan is not compelling, with those who have experienced working abroad tending to be especially aware of the peculiarly Japanese nature of this preventative approach. The position of doctors as reflexive practitioners who are also keen to maintain the ontological-security and trust of their patients exposes these professionals to tensions within their clinical work and private practices. These are in many ways consonant with the tensions experienced by the local healthcare practitioners researched by Desmond (2015) in rural Tanzania who work between two contrasting cultural-organisational configurations of risk understandings (Douglas, 1992).

Some of the underlying cultural symbols and ritual practices which underpin the risk practices of 'gargling' explored by Armstrong-Hough are further illuminated within the historical-anthropological study of Alaszewska and Alaszewski (2015). Researching the Japanese island of Aogoshima, which due to its remoteness remained relatively insulated from many of the more modern-mainstream cultural influences present within mainland Japan, a rather rich picture emerges of various more historical and enduring practices for handling the possibility of future dangers. The geo-politically significant role of the island within parts of Japanese history, alongside the unusually literate nature of some of its inhabitants in earlier centuries, presented the authors with exciting possibilities for understanding various evolving and enduring rituals and other practices for coping with uncertainty and danger – as are understood through the triangulation of ethnographic and historical-documentary data. Especially apparent within this analysis is the culturally potent symbolic connection between the health of the individual body and that of the nation, as epitomised in concerns with the well-being of the emperor. Significantly, as the relative importance of Aogoshima for the national 'body politic' has waned, so have the traditional approaches to protecting the embodied health of the local community come under threat, with those practices of divination and exorcism which endure largely focused on the individual; as importantly shaped by the Tokyo government's prohibition of these practices. The study also draws our attention to the localised variation in approaches to uncertainty and risk across national territories, as well as the manner by which social upheavals may create new possibilities for magical practices in some contexts (Desmond, 2015) or undermine these in other localities (Alaszewska & Alaszewski, 2015).

Such nuanced variations and continuities cast an uneasy light over grander narratives which link risk to distinctively new forms of modernity and cosmopolitanism, as most notably articulated by Beck (1992). The study of van Voorst (2015) develops an interrogation of four key tenets of the risk society thesis in light of her fieldwork amongst poverty-stricken, flood-prone slum districts in Jakarta, Indonesia. The analysis, developed from a rather expansive study involving ethnographic, interview and survey methods, problematises Beck's delineation of new forms of 'manufactured' risks in that flooding problems in central Jakarta have been recorded for many centuries while various human interventions would appear to be intensifying the frequency and severity of high water levels. van Voorst (2015) emphasises the importance of exploring experiences of risks more generally, rather than inquiring into specific risks, in order to identify the interconnections between different risks – in her case-study the interwovenness of poverty-related and flooding-related risks in the emic accounts of her research participants. The inextricable interaction between these 'different' risks, through which flood risks are universal in Jakarta yet experienced and coped with in highly distinct ways – as rooted in socio-economic geographies – adds important nuance to Beck's theses of risk as both democratic and universal.

Variation in approaches to uncertainty and risk within countries, let alone across global regions, is once again apparent when one compares van Voorst's (2015) study with that of Bastide (2015). While faith, especially Islamic faith, was scarcely apparent within the narratives regarding uncertainty of the urban slum-dwellers amongst which van Voorst lived, Bastide's research amongst migrants who had left Indonesian islands to travel to work in Singapore or Malaysia found that the attempts to understand and follow the will of Allah were, alongside material approaches to risk, fundamental to how many migration-related risks were handled. Amongst a number of fascinating themes explored by Bastide is the relationship between fate and agency. The agentic qualities of 'living with' or 'at' risk are usually contrasted with the passivity of fate-oriented traditional approaches to the future, in order to emphasise the nature of lived experiences which are characteristic of reflexive modernity (Beck, 1992; Giddens, 1991). Bastide (2015), meanwhile, conceptualises the dangers of migration as being confronted through 'acts of faith' – with fathoming and following the will of God involving much agency, choices, edge-work (Lyng, 2004), reflexivity and thus risk. Whereas Spinoza's claim of the remoteness of God from everyday causality would seem to be a fundamental background factor for the forming of the modern, reflexive individualised subject, the uncertainties faced by the participants in Bastide's research 'surrendered' many of their uncertainties to the will of God, but with the opacity of this will rendering new uncertainties and risks apparent. The enduring tension between fate and agency, the 'displacing' and replacing of responsibility, raises many questions germane to everyday life within a risky modernity, not least those pertaining to the 'moral economy' (Bastide, 2015) surrounding the responsibilised modern citizen-believer. Bastide further underlines the influence of neo-liberal and globalising tendencies, in the wider economy and consequently within the labour market, as defining structural features of the social-hierarchical landscape within which migrants travel and by which more marginalised groups are often especially vulnerable.

As central as Islamic faith was to the ways in which Bastide's participants handled uncertainty, their actions and narratives also indicated other rationalities besides faith-based ones. Returning to the conceptualisation of approaches to uncertainty which lie in between the traditional and modern (Desmond, 2015; c.f. Zinn, 2008), combining the magical with the techno-practical, important questions emerge as to how such syncretism takes place, the relative importance and hierarchy of different approaches and how tensions between different rationalities are experienced and (un)resolved. Coderey's (2015) ethnographic exploration of pluralist health-seeking practices in rural Myanmar grapples with these very questions, researching the use of exorcists, divination, various Buddhist devotions and biomedicine (referred to locally as 'knowledge of the English remedies') and how these were selectively drawn upon and combined. In her findings, different approaches were more or less likely to be used for different purposes – prevention, cure, understanding of the underlying aetiology – while geography, education, familiarity and (dis)trust also bore significantly on the (non-)use of synthetic 'English remedies'/pharmaceutical products. Coping with uncertainty amidst illness experiences followed different rationalities, as more or less caused by spiritual powers, for example, depending on the nature, duration and severity of these experiences. Ultimately, however, these plural approaches were understood within an underlying Buddhist cosmology – with karma, echoing Bastide's (2015) analysis of fate, existing in a tension between its deterministic qualities and its amenability to be enhanced through agency.

Rereading the handling of uncertainty within northern European post-industrial societies in light of 'different modernities'

The central themes of the articles in this special issue, as sketched above, provide a range of useful insights into exploring approaches to uncertainty (including risk) in different modernising contexts around the globe. They also raise a number of important questions for analyses of how uncertain futures are handled within northern Europe. While Desmond (2015) applies the notion of a location in between tradition and modernity to the specific context of sub-Saharan Africa, a similar conceptualisation of contexts in northern Europe could offer up a number of fruitful lines of investigation.

In his argument for a greater attentiveness towards the combining of sacred-magical and mundane-practical approaches to uncertainty, Bastide (2015) cites Favret-Saada (1977) as one of a small number of studies to have explored the magical in modern France – an intimate ethnography of enduring practices of witchcraft within one rural area in the west of the country. While these archetypal aspects of the magical continue to exist, albeit on the margins, in northern European societies, there are other ways in which notions of the sacred, magical and the ritualistic shape many ways of thinking and doing (Alaszewski, 2015) – acting as powerful rationalities in their own right as well as potential impediments to a 'rationalisation' of our socio-cultural lifeworlds (Habermas, 1987) around risk:

A sacralisation of childhood has emerged across the twentieth century (Zelizer, 1994), in contrast to the status of children in the late nineteenth century, and has become especially potent within Anglo-Saxon cultures and their mass-media driven public spheres. This tendency warps and impedes a more 'communicatively rational' approach to dealing with risk to children of harm or abuse (Alaszewski & Brown, 2012; Warner, 2015).

Alaszewski and Brown (2015), meanwhile, explore various ways in which attempts to rationalise time within organisations become obfuscated by the rituals which inevitably emerge within large organisations, even (or perhaps especially) within supposedly scientific-bureaucratic ones. Here they refer to Roth's (1957) study of American hospitals' approaches to managing the risk of Tuberculosis infection (see also Alaszewski, 2015). The enduring uncertainty around the extent of contagiousness, mode of infection and optimal mode of prevention led to norms for dealing with the disease which were based more on routine and ritual than any form of evidence-base to the extent that Roth (1957, p. 310) posits some aspects as verging on the magical.

For the participants in Coderey's (2015) study in rural Myanmar, it was the limitations of any one approach in handling the uncertainty of illness which ensured the extent of pluralistic health-seeking. Similarly, the persistent and inherent uncertainties of a scientific-bureaucratic rationality – not least around risk – leave a vacuum of 'knowing' within which the magical, religious and/or ritualistic continue to be apposite. In his review of the publication of Favret-Saada's (1977) study in English (Favret-Saada, 1980), Lewis (1981) reflected back upon Evans-Pritchard's (1937) classic study of witchcraft in central Africa (see Alaszewski, 2015 for a useful overview and re-analysis) to emphasise the benefits or even superiority of such practices – particularly in dealing with the 'why me?' questions. Unlike probabilistic approaches which help individuals understand why they are or were *more likely* to experience a particular outcome, magical practices may be far more effective at clarifying why one individual in particular suffered and not someone else who was also 'at risk'. The 'ecological prevention paradox' – by which tendencies across larger populations inevitably offer unsatisfactory guidance for individual decision making amidst uncertainty (Heyman, 2010, p. 100) – may similarly be experienced as less salient for some persons than magical or religious ways of approaching futures.

This everyday sense-making success of the magical, often embedded within the religious, is clear within Coderey's (2015) study in rural Myanmar where combinations of magical and/or religious approaches, ultimately grounded in a Buddhist cosmology, are considered to leave far fewer question marks over causality in individual cases than the biomedical. Sociological studies of risk and uncertainty have generally overlooked the role of religious faith in dealing with uncertainty and how such faith sits more or less awkwardly alongside more biomedical-based risk approaches. Key early texts within the field (Beck, 1992; Giddens, 1991) developed grand narratives about a distinctively different modernisation where lingering traditional and religious practices were generally disregarded. However religious faith is still (and in some cases increasingly) popular in many regions and households of northern Europe and the ways in which this faith functions alongside risk, hope and trust in coping with and handling uncertain futures (see Brown, De Graaf, & Hillen, 2015, p. 222; Krause, 2014; Zinn, 2008) require detailed exploration.

In many northern European contexts the greater familiarity with and system trust in biomedicine, in contrast to Coderey's (2015) Myanmar study, are likely to involve different configurations of faith, trust, hope and risk. Substantial losses of trust in biomedicine and a related tendency towards pluralist health-seeking practices around complementary and alternative medicine in North America and northern Europe nevertheless include a number of important parallels with Coderey's study (compare with Gale, 2014; Siahpush, 2000). Further differences pertain to Buddhist cosmologies contrasting greatly with Christian or Islamic theologies in relation to how the future, the self and the benevolence of external powers are understood. Even within one 'religion', individuals' faith and theology will differ markedly and this heterogeneity would need to be attended to. Such a line of research would be highly novel yet not without existing literature to draw upon; Weber's (2004) and Kierkegaard's (1957) classic studies have much to tell us about faith and futures and these two studies are, of course, especially attentive to the salience of (Calvinist) theological specificities within broader faith groups regarding how the future is understood and approached.

Even in contexts where the magical, the ritualistic or the religious have seemingly lapsed as practices and passed into history, traditions nevertheless live on as deeply implicit yet powerful cultural 'sedimentations' (Shilling, 2002). Professional and public understandings of the health-protective effects of breast-feeding, or the risk of the person diagnosed with psychosis, for example, should not be analysed without due recognition for the way deep-rooted sedimentations of traditional cultural tropes of 'natural mothering' or the demon-possessed 'mad-man' linger on (or are re-manufactured) through various symbolic, metaphorical, linguistic, conceptual and institutional legacies (Faircloth, 2013; Warner & Gabe, 2004). Where highly individualised and psychologised approaches to the risk of death have replaced earlier practices of prayer, as Seale (2002) argues is the case with hegemonic Anglo-Saxon cancer narratives, these 'modern' logics by which 'suffering produces endurance, endurance produces character and character produces hope' can nevertheless be seen to be inescapably rooted within Judeo-Christian cultural stocks-of-knowledge (Bible – English Standard Version – Romans 5: 3–4). Considerations of how these quasi-traditional cultural tropes interact with probabilities, base-rates and outcome data (Szmukler, 2003; Warner & Gabe, 2004) – within professional practice and the everyday lives of mothers, those diagnosed with psychosis or cancer patients – would take us beyond a two-dimensional account of late-modern 'rationalities' towards much richer, multi-layered and nuanced models.

Conclusion: towards an analysis of 'dealing with uncertainty and risk in everyday practice'

This editorial has sought to introduce the contents and central themes of this special issue on social theories of risk and uncertainty across a range of different modernities. Exploring manifold ways in which risks and uncertainties are handled, a number of core themes have been illuminated which represent important starting points for future research across social contexts in Asia and Africa as well as the particular form of late-modernity usually associated with northern Europe. From Malinowski's Trobriand Islanders to the various settings explored within the ethnographies within this issue, *all* approaches to uncertainty can be seen as including both magical/traditional and technical-rational or material approaches to risk (see Zinn, 2008 for a related approach). These combinations demand both more passive and agentic qualities of social actors, but in a far more nuanced manner (see Bastide, 2015) than the usual approach of linking risk to modernity and individual agency.

One recurring theme across the different articles in this issue is the logic of these combinations of various approaches to uncertainty, as especially exposed by Coderey (2015). Zinn (2008), has problematised the classic dualism of rational versus non-rational approaches to uncertainty, exploring different strategies which can be seen as comprising both more calculative and non-calculative elements. These 'in-between' strategies such as emotion, trust and intuition are vital in absorbing the residual uncertainty left by prob-abilistic risk-oriented approaches. Alongside investigation of the combinations of these different approaches for dealing with uncertainty and risk in everyday practice, this current issue has emphasised still other approaches – not least faith-based ones – which are highly salient for many social actors in (late-)modernities.

Also found in this double issue is a call for papers which encourages authors to submit articles, picking up on these latter and related themes, for consideration for the 2016 theory special issue. Of particular interest is how different approaches to uncertainty are pragmatically combined by actors in everyday settings. Past work in this journal and indeed in this issue has started to unpick such processes and logics of 'bricolage' (Horlick-Jones et al., 2007), syncretism or pluralism (see Coderey, 2015), but this remains an under-theorised topic within social-scientific accounts of risk and uncertainty. It is fitting, if also frustrating, that this topic emerges in the year following the death of Tom Horlick-Jones. Tom was a generous, insightful and prolific thinker-researcher who con-tributed a great deal to this field theoretically and empirically. His interest in pragmatic approaches to risk and uncertainty, inspired by ethnomethodology, will continue to be both significant and greatly missed. The forthcoming special issue will be worked on in memory of his writings and his friendship.

Disclosure statement

No potential conflict of interest was reported by the author.

References

Alaszewska, J., & Alaszewski, A. (2015). Purity and danger: Shamans, diviners and the control of danger in pre-modern Japan as evidenced by the healing rites of the Aogashima islanders. *Health, Risk & Society, 17*(3–4), 302–325.

Alaszewski, A. (2015). Anthropology and risk: Insights into uncertainty, danger and blame from other cultures. *Health, Risk & Society, 17*(3–4), 205–225.

Alaszewski, A., & Brown, P. (2012). *Making health policy: A critical introduction*. Cambridge: Polity.

Alaszewski, A., & Brown, P. (2015). Time, risk and health. In M. Chamberlain (Ed.), *Risk, health and discourse*. London: Routledge.

Alaszewski, A., & Burgess, A. (2007). Risk, time and reason. *Health, Risk & Society, 9*(4), 349–358. doi:10.1080/13698570701612295

Armstrong-Hough, M. (2015). Performing prevention: Risk, responsibility, and reorganising the future in Japan during the H1N1 pandemic. *Health, Risk & Society, 17*(3–4), 285–301.

Bastide, L. (2015). Faith and uncertainty: Migrants' journeys between Indonesia, Malaysia and Singapore. *Health, Risk & Society, 17*(3–4), 226–245.

Beck, U. (1992). *The risk society: Towards a new modernity*. London: Sage.

Brown, P., De Graaf, S., & Hillen, M. (2015). The inherent tensions and ambiguities of hope: Towards a post-formal analysis of experiences of advanced-cancer patients. *Health, 19*(2), 207–225.

Brubaker, R. (1984). *The limits of rationality: An essay on the social and moral thought of Max Weber*. London: Allen & Unwin.

Coderey, C. (2015). Coping with health-related uncertainties and risks in Rakhine (Myanmar). *Health, Risk & Society, 17*(3–4), 263–284.

Desmond, N. (2015). Engaging with risk in non-Western settings: An editorial. *Health, Risk & Society, 17*(3–4), 196–204.

Douglas, M. (1992). *Risk and blame: Essays in cultural theory*. London: Routledge.

Douglas, M., & Wildavsky, A. (1983). *Risk and culture: An essay on the selection of technological and environmental dangers*. Berkeley: University of California Press.

Evans-Pritchard, E. E. (1937). *Witchcraft, oracles and magic among the Azande*. Oxford: The Clarendon Press.

Faircloth, C. (2013). *Militant Lactivism? Attachment parenting and intensive motherhood in the UK and France*. Oxford: Berghahn.

Favret-Saada, J. (1977). *Les mots, la mort, les sorts*. Paris: Gallimard.

Favret-Saada, J. (1980). *Deadly words: Witchcraft in the Bocage*. Cambridge: Cambridge University Press.

Foucault, M. (1974/1994). The birth of social medicine. In J. Faubion (Ed.), *Michel Foucault – power: Essential works of Foucault 1954-1984* (Vol. 3). London: Penguin.

Gale, N. (2014). The sociology of traditional, complementary and alternative medicine. *Sociology Compass, 8*(6), 805–822. doi:10.1111/soc4.12182

Giddens, A. (1991). *Modernity and self-identity: Self and society in the late-modern age*. Cambridge: Polity.

Habermas, J. (1976). *Legitimation crisis*. Cambridge: Polity.

Habermas, J. (1987). *Theory of communicative action (vol 2): Lifeworld and system – a critique of functionalist reason*. Cambridge: Polity.

Heyman, B. (2010). Health risks and probabilistic reason. In B. Heyman, M. Shaw, A. Alaszewski, & M. Titterton (Eds.), *Risk, safety and clinical practice: Healthcare through the lens of risk*. Oxford: Oxford University Press.

Heyman, B., & Brown, P. (2013). Perspectives on the 'lens' of risk: Interview series: Interviews with Judith Green and Peter Taylor-Gooby. *Health, Risk & Society, 15*(1), 12–26. doi:10.1080/13698575.2012.755501

Horlick-Jones, T., Walls, J., & Kitzinger, J. (2007). *Bricolage* in action: Learning about, making sense of, and discussing, issues about genetically modified crops and food. *Health, Risk & Society, 9*(1), 83–103. doi:10.1080/13698570601181623

Kierkegaard, S. (1957). *The concept of dread*. New York, NY: WW Norton.

Krause, K. (2014). Pharmaceutical potentials: Praying over medicines in Pentecostal healing. *Ghana Studies, 15–16*, 223–250.

Lewis, I. (1981). Why me? Review of Favret-Saada, J. *Deadly words: Witchcraft in the Bocage. London Review of Books, 3*(11), 15–16.

Lyng, S. (2004). *Edgework: The sociology of risk taking*. London: Routledge.

Malinowski, B. (1999). *Argonauts of the Western Pacific*. London: Routledge.

Mieulet, E., & Claeys, C. (2014). The implementation and reception of policies for preventing dengue fever epidemics: A comparative study of Martinique and French Guyana. *Health, Risk & Society, 16*(7–8), 581–599. doi:10.1080/13698575.2014.949224

Mythen, G. (2007). Reappraising the risk society thesis: Telescopic sight or myopic vision? *Current Sociology, 55*(6), 793–813. doi:10.1177/0011392107081986

Ohnuki-Tierney, E. (1984). *Illness and culture in contemporary Japan.* Cambridge: Cambridge University Press.

Outhwaite, W. (2009). *Habermas: A critical introduction.* Cambridge: Polity.

Roth, J. (1957). Ritual and magic in the control of contagion. *American Sociological Review, 22*(3), 310–314. doi:10.2307/2088472

Rothstein, H. (2006). The institutional origins of risk: A new agenda for risk research. *Health, Risk & Society, 8*(3), 215–221. doi:10.1080/13698570600871646

Seale, C. (2002). Cancer heroics: A study of news reports with particular reference to gender. *Sociology, 36*(1), 107–126.

Shilling, C. (2002). Culture, the 'sick role' and the consumption of health. *British Journal of Sociology, 53*(4), 621–638. doi:10.1080/0007131022000021515

Siahpush, M. (2000). A critical review of the sociology of alternative medicine: Research on users, practitioners and the orthodoxy. *Health, 4*(2), 159–178.

Szmukler, G. (2003). Risk assessment: Numbers and values. *Psychiatric Bulletin, 27*(6), 205–207. doi:10.1192/pb.27.6.205

van Loon, J. (2013) The optics of risk: Mediatisation, anticipation and the logistics of perception. Keynote lecture: Amsterdam Risk Conference, Univeristy of Amsterdam, 23 January 2013.

van Voorst, R. (2015). Applying the risk society thesis within the context of flood risk and poverty in Jakarta, Indonesia. *Health, Risk & Society, 17*(3–4), 246–262.

Warner, J. (2015). *The emotional politics of social work and child protection.* Bristol: Policy Press.

Warner, J., & Gabe, J. (2004). Risk and liminality in mental health social work. *Health, Risk & Society, 6*(4), 387–399. doi:10.1080/13698570412331323261

Watt, A. (1972). The causality of God in Spinoza's philosophy. *Canadian Journal of Philosophy, 2*(2), 171–189.

Weber, M. (2004). *The protestant ethic and the 'Spirit' of capitalism.* London: Penguin.

Wilkinson, I. (2010). *Risk, vulnerability and everyday life.* London: Routledge.

Zelizer, V. (1994). *Pricing the priceless child: The changing social value of children.* New Jersey, NJ: Princeton University Press.

Zinn, J. (2008). Heading into the unknown: Everyday strategies for managing risk and uncertainty. *Health, Risk & Society, 10*(5), 439–450. doi:10.1080/13698570802380891

Engaging with risk in non-Western settings: an editorial

Nicola Desmond

In this guest editorial I argue for the need to resituate an understanding of risk perception within linguistic and methodological frameworks across different cultural settings. Drawing on long-term ethnographic fieldwork in north-western Tanzania, I briefly explore the concept of risk as it has evolved in Western settings from post-Enlightenment scientific tradition. I question the underlying assumptions of Western scientific notions of risk and consider the concepts of risk and uncertainty as they relate to broader social discourses of modernity, tradition, development and social change within a postcolonial sub-Saharan Africa setting. Acknowledging but moving beyond the social framing of risk put forward by Mary Douglas and others including Deborah Lupton and Pat Caplan, and following Jens Zinn in proposing the need for a refined notion of risk, I argue that the influence of language and method is intrinsic to the ways we conceptualise and subjectivise risk. Drawing on research exploring the risk perceptions of actors engaged in health prevention in a non-Western setting in Tanzania – those of externally funded health interventions, government biomedical service providers and local, lay populations – I show how framing of what is considered a priority for health is culturally contingent. Further I suggest that this cultural contingency is reproduced in encounters with researchers, framing risk according to broader social circumstance and situated dynamically within the context of people's everyday life experiences. This necessitates a process of refinement which is only likely to be achieved under certain conditions; if emic categories are taken into account, if the complexity and contingency of risk and its interpretation is acknowledged through language and if there is greater recognition and awareness of the direct impact of method on individual risk prioritisation and framing, moving towards a more ethnographic approach to go beyond superficial understandings and explore the tensions between what people say they do and what they actually do. These conditions for enhancing engagement with risk become more important given an increasingly influential globalisation; creating a dynamic social world in sub-Saharan Africa, in which risk priorities are constantly reassessed and management strategies renegotiated as individuals encounter novel and changing lifeworlds.

Introduction

In this guest editorial, I explore the methodological and linguistic realities of engaging with the concept of risk in health through ethnography within the non-Western setting of Tanzania in sub-Saharan Africa. Drawing on several years of ethnographic engagement, I explore the concepts of risk and uncertainty as they relate to broader social discourses of modernity, tradition, development and social change and the impact of linguistic and methodological framing on our understanding of risk perception.

Risk and health

Risk as a conceptual category has been the subject of much discussion in the sociology of health in recent years but there remain significant differences in the way it is framed and defined (Henwood, Pidgeon, Sarre, Simmons, & Smith, 2008). Researchers have focused on understanding how risk should be considered in the light of its relevance to other aspects of people's lives (Fischoff, 1985; Lupton & Tulloch, 2002a, 2002b) and others have argued that it is only a relevant concept where there is choice of alternative lifestyles (Beck, 1992; Giddens, 1990, 1991). Yet others have suggested that risk is contingent, either on social position and 'cultural biases' (Douglas, 1985, 1992; Douglas & Wildavsky, 1982) or as expert knowledge (Giddens, 1991, 1994). These theories are drawn from and in turn contribute to a Western conceptualisation of risk perception; one that is progressive, evidence-based and rational and situated historically and socially within a post-Enlightenment tradition of modernity, postmodernity and development discourse. Western biomedical approaches to health risk have been and continue to be informed by this progressive, scientific paradigm underpinned by an unchallenged assumption of objectivity.

Risk in sub-Saharan Africa

As an anthropologist working largely within sub-Saharan Africa, I have engaged with the concept of risk predominantly in non-Western settings and often situated within the framework of uncertainty (Boholm, 1996; Rosa, 2003; Whyte, 1997). This has led me to question some of the underlying premises in the historical framing of risk as a construct of post-Enlightenment Western thought and its applicability to non-Western settings. Foucault argued that the historical context and particularly its shaping of what is possible, of what can be seen, determines what at any time is considered to be true (Foucault, 1973). Understanding of risk has not developed in sub-Saharan Africa within the same historical trajectory as that of the West, although it has been influenced by a series of historical phases of 'empire' including colonialism, postcolonialism and neocolonialism through a discourse of development and aid. Risk in today's non-Western setting of sub-Saharan Africa has been primarily 'claimed' by the HIV world as a heuristic behavioural concept that exists to be overcome or minimised, although it has also been deconstructed by several anthropologists working in this area (see, for example, Bujra, 2000; Dilger, 2003; Setel, 1999). There have been many studies on the nature of risk perception as well as on the embedded nature of risk behaviour (Coates, Richter, & Caceres, 2008), either within a discourse of poverty, structural violence and inequality (Barnett & Whiteside, 2002, Farmer, Lindenbaum, & Good, 1993; Lockhart, 2008; Seidel, 1993) or one of broader social (Bloor 1995; Dilger, 2003; Smith & Watkins, 2005; Swidler & Watkins, 2007) or cultural (Obbo, 1995) forces and wider social consequences of foregrounding one particular risk (Schoepf, 1995; Setel, 1996; Smith, 2003; Wallman, 2000). Its place within a broader reflection on behaviour has been taken by the construct of uncertainty, which has dominated debate in non-Western settings. This has been partly informed by a belief that risk is a modern concept and only relevant under conditions of choice and thus contingency or that risk gains in popularity as societies 'progress' from the traditional to modernity. In contrast, Africanist literature would suggest that dichotomising tradition and modernity is inappropriate in non-Western contexts (Appadurai, 1996; Karp & Masolo, 2000). Uncertainty may be directed towards the future, but has evolved in the Africanist literature as a concept explaining misfortune, not predicting it and is therefore passive rather than active. In this framing, the event may have occurred but the cause of that event may still remain uncertain and multiple causes may be attributed (Douglas, 1990). This explains a historical preference for uncertainty over risk amongst anthropologists, particularly when considering schools of functionalism and structural functionalism embedded within colonial discourses (for example, Evans-Pritchard and Radcliffe-Brown from the 1930s to 1960s) and the seeking of explanation for misfortune as dominant over seeking to avoid misfortune. More recently uncertainty has been linked more closely to risk in the sub-Saharan African literature within anthropology (Einarsdottir, 2005; Geissler, 2005), particularly in relation to globalisation and as people are increasingly exposed to expanding social lives inviting greater possibilities and choices and in so doing, introducing greater opportunity to recognise, prioritise and manage risk as a preventive construct.

My research in sub-Saharan Africa over many years has led me to interrogate the notion and utility of risk as a concept in non-Western contexts, initially from the perspective of HIV but increasingly as an overarching framework for interpreting and situating behaviour, albeit embedded within social structures less amenable to change. Here I want to explore two main aspects of the application of risk within non-Western settings, both of which are rarely understood. Firstly, I interrogate the linguistic relevance of risk and whether this term is sufficient to capture the complexity of indigenous or emic concepts of 'risk' (Allen, 2002) in contemporary sub-Saharan Africa. Secondly, and acknowledging the methodological cross-disciplinarity between sociology and anthropology of my research on risk, I also address the relationship between method and risk perception, moving on from Tulloch and Lupton's argument that risk must be understood within the context of everyday lives in their deductive approach to exploring the relevance of Beck's Risk Society thesis (Lupton & Tulloch, 2002a, 2002b), to explore examples of differing risk priorities emphasised according to methodological approach. Whilst it is widely acknowledged that risk is a cross-disciplinary research area, and thus one that can be explored from the perspective of, for example, individual psychology, economics or mathematics, the intra-disciplinarity of risk as a research theme is the subject of much less debate in the literature. This is something that I raise as an area for future research, arguing that greater attention should be paid to the method itself, both in defining what is considered risky by people at particular times and how these definitions then inform individualised risk management strategies.

The linguistic relevance of risk in sub-Saharan Africa

My work across cultural and linguistic contexts has highlighted the need to ensure collective, local meaning of terms are clear when discussing risk. My starting point for risk during research in rural and peri-urban areas of north-western Tanzania was 'the likelihood or possibility of danger'; in other words, a concept that combines both negative outcome with likelihood of occurrence and one that was drawn very much from a Western paradigm. I quickly realised, however, the need to develop a 'thick description' (Geertz, 1973) of risk, exploring local meaning and identifying the subtleties of terms which may highlight culturally relevant concepts of risk that are difficult to translate. Working in East Africa, the Swahili term *hatari* was my starting point. And indeed this was the most commonly used emic term to describe 'risk'. Other frequently used terms included words that could be translated as: 'to expose something to danger', often unwillingly. These were applied for example in discussions about sending children away from parental control to study where they may instead choose to abandon their studies and lose their own and their parents opportunity to attain a different future. Another term could be translated as 'to take a chance'. The connotations of this 'chance taking' are noteworthy since they imply active risk-taking rather than passive exposure to risk and, in areas where farming dominated livelihood strategies, such terms were readily invoked in discussions around agriculture and the need to ensure crop success given unpredictable and fluctuating weather conditions – suggesting that, whilst rainfall was unpredictable, the risk was worth taking, partly because there was no alternative to reliance on subsistence farming.

Four other terms were commonplace within emic framings of risk, each of which related to particular types of risky situation. The word *wasiwasi* was used regularly to describe 'anxiety' or 'misgivings' often to describe anxieties about exposure to the jealousy of others and often used in relation to HIV. Alternatively *mashaka* translated to 'worries', 'fear' or 'concerns' and was used to describe fears of future negative outcomes of current uncontrollable conditions, such as those pertaining to potential accusations of witchcraft or fear of insufficient food following periods of drought. The word *madhara*, translated directly as 'violence', 'loss', 'hurt' or 'injury' was also in common usage when describing the negative outcome of 'risky' behaviour, such as the social segregation of individuals who have inflicted hurt or loss in communities through theft or witchcraft. Finally, the term *balaa* was used specifically to describe 'misfortune' related to witchcraft. Commonly this was applied to descriptions of events for which the cause was unknown but the generalised implication was the influence of malevolence through sorcery or witchcraft, more so when the damage inflicted was targeted at the whole community rather than at individuals.

Whilst I acknowledge that the Swahili terms will not be familiar to many readers, I have included them here to highlight the context-driven nature of risk perceptions. What underpins these terms and their applications is the relationship between risk and misfortune where risk describes a future-oriented expectation of an event whilst misfortune describes an event that has already occurred. Whilst Giddens has argued that risk is only negotiable in a 'late modern world' in which people have diverse choices (Giddens, 1991), this brief exploration of vernacular risk terms highlights the interconnectedness of risk and misfortune, especially in many non-Western societies situated between the two worlds of tradition and modernity. People's strategies of thinking about risk in the future, in these contexts, are often deeply influenced by what has happened in the past. This approach has produced a continuum of ideas rooted in experience and re-produced in the present to influence the future and has provided traditional healers and indeed, witches, with a continued role in society's transitioning state from tradition-based to those drawing influences from wider processes and exposures to modern and often, global systems. Witchcraft in historical Africanist ethnography was an intrinsic element of social relations whilst in European historical anthropology it was considered part of processes of social change (Macfarlane & Sharpe, 1999). Reflecting more closely this European usage, witchcraft has been described in modern sub-Saharan Africa as a discourse in the search for meaning and as a response to uncertainty, for example in South Africa (Ashforth, 2002) and Zimbabwe (Rodlach, 2006). Rather than an outdated and disappearing artefact of tradition, it has instead become adaptive to the conditions of social change in contemporary sub-Saharan Africa, able to reinvent itself precisely because of its ambivalent and dynamic status (Geshiere, 1997) and it is increasingly viewed as a response to the uncertainty brought about by development (Comaroff & Comaroff, 1999). I use the example of witchcraft here to emphasise the framing of risk discourse within non-Western settings today. It highlights the development of an African modernity that can be defined as a reinvention of traditions (Hobsbawn & Ranger, 1983) and continuity with the past. In contrast, modernity in Western settings is rather described as a post-traditional state and one that facilitates the concept of risk because of the increase in lifestyle opportunities it entails. But a linguistic exploration of terms used to describe risk in a non-Western setting highlights this continuity over the disconnect.

Implications of methodologies for understanding risk

Understanding an emic perspective on risk in non-Western settings would not have been possible without adopting an ethnographic method to the study of risk perception. In this observation I am not suggesting anything novel, indeed, Caplan (2000) described the need to create 'an ethnographic method which considers risk in particular times and places and through the voices of particular informants', one that 'sees individuals in their social context, as embedded in networks of relationships which have an important bearing on their perceptions of risk' (Caplan, 2000). Our understanding of the salience of a particular risk in individual lives or how people rank the risks they feel they are exposed to and their perceived ability or willingness to pursue particular risk management strategies is necessarily influenced by the type of method we choose to investigate risk, in other words, by issues of framing (Henwood et al., 2008; Lupton, 1999). These issues of framing go beyond the context of the study setting to a broader political context of funding, instrumental in defining research priorities today. Whilst early twentieth century anthropological research was in many ways, a disinterested endeavour, conducting fieldwork for its own ends, field research in sub-Saharan Africa today is influenced by a broader global, public health discourse to address large-scale social problems such as HIV/AIDS. This has influenced a transition in contemporary African ethnography from a focus on uncertainty to one foregrounding risk and disembedding 'risky behaviour' from its wider social context. My experience in sub-Saharan Africa emphasises the importance of re-embedding an approach to understanding risk within this broader social setting, reframing risk as a situated experience (Bostrom & Desmond, 2014). Research exploring the lives and perspectives of individuals on risk and uncertainty, identified a greater number of risks discussed when embedded in informal discussion and in life history narratives than those raised when risk is considered as an abstract concept, removed from its social context (Desmond, 2009). This is likely to relate to the fact, as Tulloch and Lupton (2003) have observed that risk as an abstract category is a challenging concept to consider and most people find any abstract reflections on their life fairly challenging (Lupton & Tulloch, 2002a, 2002b).

To explore this relationship between method and perception further I will focus briefly on the risk perceptions of two groups of actors engaged in health prevention in a non-Western setting in Tanzania. I spent a period of seven years in the Mwanza Region of north-western Tanzania during which I conducted research to identify the risks considered salient to people across both a rural and peri-urban setting and to explore perceptions of and discourses influencing this salience. The approach balanced a deductive testing of the theories of Douglas and Giddens with the inductive development of new meso-theory (Hart, 1999), grounded in the research data. The former was dependent on more structured sampling and methods whilst the latter relied on a more flexible approach whilst benefiting from the tools of the former. This approach enabled me to explore how perceptions of health priorities contrast between externally funded health interventions and government biomedical service providers and how this differs from local, lay populations. I suggest that risk perception at each of these levels is culturally contingent, framed by context and arising out of culture (Douglas &

Wildavsky, 1982), each culture providing a partial perspective on the local risk landscape, strengthening Douglas' perspective, described by Boyne (2003), that 'which risks, at which level, are acceptable to which groups of people is always a social question' (Boyne, 2003). Whilst it is usually more acceptable to view emic or lay perspectives of risk as contingent on wider discourses, I suggest that risk is also constructed and made meaningful by professional bodies (researchers or biomedical providers), aligned to externally driven priorities and emergent organisational cultures.

In the former case of external health interventions, funding priorities help to inform and define a socially constructed 'objectivity' in risk perception where the intention of the health intervention clearly reflects wider funding trends and wider discourses which are situated within a politically informed narrative of risk that is created and made relevant by Western policymakers. This fails to reflect either the health risk priorities for health experienced by the lay population or key causes of mortality and morbidity perceived by local government biomedical services. Local biomedical services risk assessments are no less value-laden and partial accounts of the risk landscape. The main health problem identified by health service providers was malaria across all age groups, with diagnosis dependent primarily on symptom presentation with little clinical examination. Biomedical personnel were keen to demonstrate their 'medical objectivity' but also emphasised the constraints they faced in accurate and consistent diagnosis and whilst they did not directly admit they made errors, this very recognition of the constraints they faced (such as lack of access to laboratory facilities) provided evidence of their own partiality and subjectivities. This partiality was influenced by the fact that the biomedical providers were situated between the two worlds of risk definitions, that of biomedicine and that of the local, lay community of which they were respected members, subject to the same codes of meaning as the population they served. This contradiction was most clearly evidenced in the disparities between service providers' reported and actual action. The illness described as *mchango* provides one of the clearest examples of this contradiction (Desmond, Prost, & Wight, 2012). In local explanatory models, this is a Swahili term, directly translated as 'intestinal worms'. It is distinguished by its invisibility to biomedical tests, though it can be diagnosed through divination. Injections and biomedical treatment of the symptoms are believed to result in death. Through such risk perceptions this illness is 'protected' from the intervention of biomedicine. This invisibility inevitably must place doubt on the existence of *mchango* amongst biomedically trained health workers. And in reported perceptions and practice, it is described by health personnel as lay fallacy. In actual practice, however, *mchango* is a daily reality faced by health workers and there was in place a regular, though informal, referral system between the health centre and a local traditional healer, renowned for her skills in the recognition and treatment of *mchango*. Thus, whilst health workers conformed to expected norms of biomedical learning and experience in their discourse, their daily realities and their position as members of the community forced them to engage daily more syncretic approaches and the contradictions these gave rise to.

These examples demonstrate the partiality of risk perspectives and how each is informed by unique interpretations of the wider social environment. Whether this be funding trends and epidemiologically assessed health problems on a global or national scale or contradictory social and professional roles of local service providers under service capacity constraints. They also show, along with my consideration of linguistic interpretations of risk, how risk perception should be addressed in context and as embodied through experience (Bourdieu, 1980), particularly in non-Western settings.

Conclusion

Regardless of its origins in Western scientific traditions, risk is becoming an increasingly important concept in unpacking complex social worlds in sub-Saharan Africa today. But ground remains to be covered, particularly in unpacking concepts of risk-taking and risk acceptability, both in understanding responses, particularly those of young people, to risks of HIV under novel conditions of accessible, biomedical treatments for prevention, and equally importantly, in understanding of broader responses to health risks. Green (2009) questions whether the category of risk continues to serve an empirical purpose in determining how individuals respond to health (Green, 2009). Her suggested solution is to consider abandoning the concept completely due to its reductionist status. In many ways this may be true in non-Western settings where the term has been limited in scope due to its association, especially within biomedical frameworks, with an objectifiable reality. However I would argue, following Zinn (2009) that instead of discarding the term altogether, the concept of risk should be 'refined and developed'. This process of refinement is likely to be achieved under certain conditions; if emic categories are taken into account, if the complexity and contingency of risk and its interpretation is acknowledged through language and if there is greater recognition and awareness of the direct impact of method on individual risk prioritisation and framing moving towards a more ethnographic approach to go beyond superficial understandings and explore the tensions between what people say they do and what they actually do. These conditions for enhancing our engagement with the concept of risk become more important given an increasingly influential globalisation; creating a dynamic social world in sub-Saharan Africa, in which risk priorities are constantly reassessed and management strategies renegotiated as individuals encounter novel and changing lifeworlds.

References

Allen, D. R. (2002). *Managing motherhood, managing risk: Fertility and danger in West Central Tanzania*. Ann Arbor: University of Michigan Press.

Appadurai, A. (1996). *Modernity at large: Cultural dimensions of globalization*. Minneapolis: University of Minnesota Press.

Ashforth, A. (2002). An epidemic of witchcraft? The implications of AIDS for the post-apartheid state. *African Studies*, *61*(1), 121–143. doi:10.1080/00020180220140109

Barnett, T., & Whiteside, A. (2002). *AIDS in the twenty-first century: Disease and globalization*. Basingstoke: Palgrave Macmillan.

Beck, U. (1992). *Risk society: Towards a new modernity*. London: Sage.

Bloor, M. (1995). A user's guide to contrasting theories of HIV-related risk behaviour. In J. Gabe (Ed.), *Medicine, health and risk*. Oxford: Blackwell.

Boholm, A. (1996). Risk perception and social anthropology: Critique of cultural theory. *Ethnos*, *61*(1–2), 64–84. doi:10.1080/00141844.1996.9981528

Bostrom, M., & Desmond, N. (2014). Through the rabbit hole: Considering the situational experience of risk among men who have sex with men in the context of HIV prevention. *AIDS Research and Human Retroviruses*, *30*(Suppl 1), A22–A22.

Bourdieu, P. (1980). *The logic of practice*. Stanford, CA: Stanford University Press.

Boyne, R. (2003). *Risk*. Buckingham: Open University Press.

Bujra, J. (2000). Risk and trust: Unsafe sex, gender and AIDS in Tanzania. In P. Caplan (Ed.), *Risk revisited*. London: Pluto Press.

Caplan, P. (2000). Introduction. In P. Caplan (Ed.), *Risk revisited*. London: Pluto Press.

Coates, T. J., Richter, L., & Caceres, C. (2008). Behavioural strategies to reduce HIV transmission: How to make them work better. *The Lancet*, *372*, 669–684. doi:10.1016/S0140-6736(08)60886-7

Comaroff, J., & Comaroff, J. L. (1999). Occult economies and the violence of abstraction: Notes from the South African postcolony. *American Ethnologist*, *26*(2), 279–303. doi:10.1525/ae.1999.26.2.279

Desmond, N. A. (2009). *'Ni kubahatisha tu!' 'It's just a game of chance!' Adaptation and resignation to perceived risks in rural Tanzania* (PhD thesis). University of Glasgow.

Desmond, N. A., Prost, A., & Wight, D. (2012). Managing risk through treatment-seeking in rural north-western Tanzania: Categorising health problems as malaria and nzoka. *Health, Risk & Society*, *14*(2), 149–170. doi:10.1080/13698575.2012.661042

Dilger, H. (2003). Sexuality, AIDS, and the lures of modernity: Reflexivity and morality among young people in rural Tanzania. *Medical Anthropology*, *22*, 23–52. doi:10.1080/01459740306768

Douglas, M. (1985). *Risk acceptability according to the social sciences*. New York, NY: Russell Sage.

Douglas, M. (1990). Risk as a forensic resource. *Daedalus*, *119*(4), 1–16.

Douglas, M. (1992). *Risk and blame: Essays in cultural theory*. London: Routledge.

Douglas, M., & Wildavsky, A. (1982). *Risk and culture: An essay on the selection of environmental and technological dangers*. Berkeley: University of California Press.

Einarsdottir, J. (2005). Restoration of social order through the extinction of non-human children. In V. Steffen, R. Jenkins, & H. Jessen (Eds.), *Managing uncertainty: Ethnographic studies of illness, risk and the struggle for control*. Copenhagen: Museum Tusculanum Press.

Farmer, P., Lindenbaum, S., & Good, M.-J. D. (1993). Women, poverty and AIDS: An introduction. *Culture Medicine and Psychiatry: An International Journal of Comparative Cross-Cultural Research*, *17*, 387–397. doi:10.1007/BF01379306

Fischoff, B. (1985). Managing risk perceptions. *Issues in Science and Technology*, *2*(1), 83–96.

Foucault, M. (1973). *The birth of the clinic*. London: Tavistock.

Geertz, C. (1973). Thick description: Toward an interpretive theory of culture. In C. Geertz (Eds.), *The interpretation of cultures*. New York, NY: Basic Books.

Geissler, W. (2005). Blood stealing rumours in Western Kenya. In R. Jenkins, H. Jessen, & V. Steffen (Eds.), *Managing uncertainty: Ethnographic studies of illness, risk and the struggle for control*. Copenhagen: Museum Tusculanum Press.

Geshiere, P. (1997). *The modernity of witchcraft: Politics and the occult in postcolonial Africa*. Charlottesville: University of Virginia Press.

Giddens, A. (1990). *The consequences of modernity*. Cambridge: Polity Press.

Giddens, A. (1991). *Modernity and self-identity: Self and society in the late modern age*. London: Polity Press.

Giddens, A. (1994). Living in a post-traditional society. In U. Beck, A. Giddens, & S. Lash (Eds.), *Reflexive modernisation*. Cambridge: Polity Press.

Green, J. (2009). Is it time for the sociology of health to abandon risk? *Health, Risk & Society*, *11*(6), 493–508. doi:10.1080/13698570903329474

Hart, G. (1999). Guest editorial: Risk and health: Challenges and opportunity. *Health, Risk & Society*, *1*(1), 7–10. doi:10.1080/13698579908407003

Henwood, K., Pidgeon, N., Sarre, S., Simmons, P., & Smith, N. (2008). Risk, framing and everyday life: Epistemological and methodological reflections from three socio-cultural projects. *Health, Risk & Society*, *10*(5), 421–438. doi:10.1080/13698570802381451

Hobsbawn, E., & Ranger, T. (Eds.). (1983). *The invention of tradition*. Cambridge: Cambridge University Press.

Karp, I., & Masolo, D. A. (Eds.). (2000). *African philosophy as cultural inquiry*. Bloomington: Indiana University Press.

Lockhart, C. (2008). The life and death of a street boy in East Africa: Everyday violence in the time of AIDS. *Medical Anthropology Quarterly*, *22*(1), 94–115. doi:10.1111/j.1548-1387.2008.00005.x

Lupton, D. (Ed.). (1999). Introduction: Risk and sociocultural theory. In *Risk and sociocultural theory: New directions and perspectives*. Cambridge: Cambridge University Press.

Lupton, D., & Tulloch, J. (2002a). 'Life would be pretty dull without risk': Voluntary risk-taking and its pleasures. *Health, Risk & Society*, *4*(2), 113–124. doi:10.1080/13698570220137015

Lupton, D., & Tulloch, J. (2002b). 'Risk is part of your life': Risk epistemologies among a group of Australians. *Sociology*, *36*, 317–334. doi:10.1177/0038038502036002005

Macfarlane, A., & Sharpe, J. A. (1999). *Witchcraft in Tudor and Stuart England: A regional and comparative study.* Oxford: Psychology Press, Routledge.

Obbo, C. (1995). Gender, age and class: Discourses on HIV transmission and control in Uganda. In H. T. Brummelhuis & G. Herdt (Eds.), *Culture and sexual risk: Anthropological perspectives on AIDS.* London: Routledge.

Rodlach, A. (2006). *Witches, Westerners and HIV: AIDS and cultures of blame in Africa.* Walnut Creek, CA: Left Coast Press.

Rosa, E. A. (2003). The logical structure of the social amplification of risk framework (SARF): Metatheoretical foundations and policy implications. In N. F. Pidgeon, R. K. Kasperson, & P. Slovic (Eds.), *The social amplification of risk.* Cambridge: Cambridge University Press.

Schoepf, B. G. (1995). Culture, sex research and AIDS prevention in Africa. In H. T. Brummelhuis & G. Herdt (Eds.), *Culture and sexual risk: Anthropological perspectives on AIDS.* London: Routledge.

Seidel, G. (1993). Women at risk: Gender and AIDS in Africa. *Disasters, 17*(2), 133–142. doi:10.1111/disa.1993.17.issue-2

Setel, P. (1996). AIDS as a paradox of manhood and development in Kilimanjaro, Tanzania. *Social Science & Medicine, 43*(8), 1169–1178. doi:10.1016/0277-9536(95)00360-6

Setel, P. (1999). *A plague of paradoxes: AIDS, culture and demography in Northern Tanzania.* Chicago, IL: The University of Chicago Press.

Smith, D. J. (2003). Imagining HIV/AIDS: Morality and perceptions of personal risk in Nigeria. *Medical Anthropology, 22*(4), 343–372. doi:10.1080/714966301

Smith, K. P., & Watkins, S. C. (2005). Perceptions of risk and strategies for prevention: Responses to HIV/AIDS in rural Malawi. *Social Science & Medicine, 60,* 649–660. doi:10.1016/j.socscimed.2004.06.009

Swidler, A., & Watkins, S. C. (2007). Ties of dependence: AIDS and transactional sex in rural Malawi. *Studies in Family Planning, 38*(3), 147–162. doi:10.1111/sifp.2007.38.issue-3

Tulloch, J., & Lupton, D. (2003). *Risk and everyday life.* London: Sage.

Wallman, S. (2000). Risk, STD and HIV infection in Kampala. *Health, Risk & Society, 2*(2), 189–203. doi:10.1080/713670157

Whyte, S. (1997). *Questioning misfortune: The pragmatics uncertainty in Eastern Uganda.* Cambridge: Cambridge University Press.

Zinn, J. (2009). The sociology of risk and uncertainty: A response to Judith Green's 'Is it time for the sociology of health to abandon "risk"?'. *Health, Risk & Society, 11*(6), 509–526. doi:10.1080/13698570903329490

Anthropology and risk: insights into uncertainty, danger and blame from other cultures: a review essay

Andy Alaszewski

In this review, I examine the contribution of social anthropology to the study of risk. I define social anthropology as the study of 'other cultures' and note that such studies have a long history, for example the Greeks and Romans were interested in exploring and understanding 'barbarians' and using such studies to reflect on their own society. However, in the early twentieth century, with the Cambridge Expedition to the Torres Straits and Malinowski's fieldwork in the Trobriand Islands, the study of other cultures shifted from an assumption of western cultural superiority to respect for other cultures with anthropologists seeking to understand and explain the unique logic and rationality of different cultures. This new approach to other cultures tended to stress the universality of the challenges which societies face while documenting their unique responses. Thus, all societies have to cope with uncertainty, the essential unpredictability of the future and account for past misfortunes. In western societies, risk now plays a central role in making the future more predictable and manageable and enabling the forensic investigation of the past. For example, in the area of health, epidemiologists map the incidence of disease and their spatial, temporal and social distribution providing a way of predicting and preventing future incidence. In other cultures, various forms of divination and ritual activity perform the same function. For example, Malinowski identified the importance of dangerous long sea journeys for the Trobriand Islanders and examined the ways in which they sought to deal with these dangers through a combination of technical skill and magic. Douglas used historical and anthropological evidence to develop a cultural theory of risk. She argued that the nature of social relations in a group influenced which hazards that group chose to highlight and sought to counteract, and how they chose to do this. Although it is possible to identify issues of risk and uncertainty in anthropological studies, it has not been a central or major theme and the contribution of anthropology to risk studies has been more limited than the contribution of disciplines such as sociology and psychology. Part of the problem relates to globalisation. The development of anthropology as a mature discipline at the end of the nineteenth century, one which respected other cultures, coincided with the peak of European colonisation. While social anthropologists wanted to explore and understand 'pristine' pre-modern cultures, the reality was that these cultures were already being reshaped by European institutions such as hospitals and medicine. In terms of uncertainty, this means that pre-modern systems of predicting and managing the future, such as oracle and magic, coexist and compete with global systems such as risk-based medicine. It is possible to recover and reconstruct such pre-modern systems by using historical sources. However, most contemporary ethnographies must take into account competing systems and how individuals choose and move between them.

Introduction

In this review, I examine the ways in which social anthropology has contributed to our understanding of the relationship between risk and society. For the purposes of this review, I use Beattie's (1964) definition of social anthropology as the study of 'other cultures'.

Development of anthropology

In Europe, curiosity about and commentary on 'other cultures' can be traced back to the classic Greek and Roman periods. Such interest was refracted through the cultural prism of the moral and military superiority of the 'civilised' Greek and Roman elites and their interactions with uncivilised, disorderly and dangerous Barbarians. For example, in his accounts of his campaigns in Gaul and Britain, Julius Caesar provided brief accounts of politics, social structures and religion, including an account of the Druids, of the Gallic tribes he was conquering and civilising (Caesar, 1996, 6.11–20). Similarly, Tacitus used his account of Boudicca's uprising in Britain to contrast civilised Romans with Barbarian Britons. In his account, the military discipline of the Roman army saved Rome from a major defeat caused by the corruption and decadence of Emperor Nero and the imperial court. The 'noble British' barbarians justly sought to avenge the Roman violation of Boudicca and her daughters but their bravery could not compensate for their individualistic and disorderly fighting tactics (Tacitus, n.d., Book XIV, Chapters 29–37).

The expansion of European states after the late fifteenth century increased contact between Europeans and other cultures and European accounts of these cultures. These accounts came from different sources, including conquerors, missionaries, explorers and adventurers. These accounts were used by intellectuals to reflect on the nature of other cultures and their relations with Europe. As Hart points out, in the eighteenth century, thinkers such as Rousseau followed Tacitus' lead, using these accounts to reflect on what civilised but corrupted Europeans could learn from primitive people living close to a state of nature. In the nineteenth century, the emphasis shifted to the Caesar's approach focussing on the racial and social evolution that accounted for the ease with which Europeans could conquer and dominate other cultures:

> The question Victorians asked was how they were able to conquer the planet with so little effective resistance. They concluded that their culture was superior, being based on reason rather than superstition, and that this superiority was grounded in nature as racial difference. (Hart, 1999, p. 1)

This assumption of superiority and the emphasis on evolution underpinned nineteenth century anthropological theorising. Frazer provided a good example of such armchair theorising. In the Golden Bough, first published in 1890, he provided an overview of pre-modern belief systems in which he claimed to show that human culture had evolved through three stages, the magical, the religious and the modern scientific. In his analysis of magic, Frazer argued that it operated in one of two ways, either through the principle that like produces like or the principle that contact between two objects creates an enduring link between them. He argued that magic is a false science based on irrationality and the magician is a doer not a thinker who is incapable of abstract logical thought:

In short, magic is a spurious system of natural law as well as a fallacious guide of conduct; it is a false science as well as an abortive art... With him [the magician], as with the vast majority of men, logic is implicit, not explicit: he reasons just as he digests his food in complete ignorance of the intellectual and physiological processes which are essential to the one operation and to the other. In short, to him magic is always an art, never a science; the very idea of science is lacking in his undeveloped mind. (Frazer, n.d., Chapter 3, section 1)

At the end of the nineteenth century, there was a major shift in both the methods and the underlying assumptions of social anthropology. The armchair theorising of Frazer based on reading of classic texts and correspondence with missionaries and others was replaced, especially in Britain, by ethnographic fieldwork. In 1898, a multi-disciplinary University of Cambridge team led by Haddon visited the Torres Straits Islands, which are politically part of Australia but culturally had more in common with Papua/New Guinea (Herle & Rouse, 1998). Haddon wanted to record the Islanders' culture before it was destroyed by zealous Christian missionaries. To this end, the team collected cultural artefacts recording the ways they were used. Not only did the team publish accounts of the Islanders culture, they also produced the earliest ethnographic films some of which have survived.

Haddon and his colleagues moved anthropology out of the armchair into the field but they were still operating within the Victorian evolutionary framework. From 1915 onwards, Malinowski developed modern ethnographic fieldwork and shifted the basic paradigm of anthropology. Malinowski was an Austro-Hungarian Pole who came to London School of Economics in 1910 to study anthropology. Initially, he did 'armchair' research but in 1914 had the opportunity to go on a field trip to New Guinea. While he was there, the First World War started so as a foreign alien he was unable to return to the UK. The Australian Government agreed that he could stay and do fieldwork in their territory and he decided to work in the Trobriand Islands, a Melanesian archipelago north of Papua/New Guinea. His enforced stay meant that he had time to learn the local language, build up a network of informants and observe and participate in Islander life and activities. When he returned to the UK after the War, he wrote a series of ethnographic studies starting in 1922 with the *Argonauts of the Western Pacific* (Malinowski, 1999).

In Malinowski's ethnography, there is a major shift in perspective. He did not look down from a position of western superiority; the disorder, carnage and barbarity of the First World War and subsequent events clearly undermined such a position. Indeed, the ethnographic method he described involved distancing himself from other westerners and learning how to behave correctly and respectfully within the host culture:

the secret of effective field-work... by which he [the ethnographer] is able to evoke the real spirit of the natives, the true picture of tribal life...consists mainly in cutting oneself of from the company of other white men, and remaining in as close contact with the natives as possible ... by means of this natural intercourse, you learn to know him, and you become familiar with his customs and beliefs... I had to learn how to behave, and to a certain extent, I acquired 'the feeling' for native good and bad manners. (Malinowski, 1999, p. 5–6)

Malinowski presented the Islanders as rational individuals who created and used social institutions and technologies to create and maintain an ordered stable society. Thus, Malinowski shifted anthropology from a system that classified societies according to an evolutionary hierarchy, to a series of case studies based on ethnographic fieldwork that examined how different social groups found their own solution to the basic challenges of living together. Hart has noted that this paradigm has dominated anthropology, especially British anthropology for most of the twentieth century:

> In the 20th century anthropology took the predominant form of ethnography. That is, individual peoples, studied in isolation from their wider context in time and space, were written up by lone ethnographers whose method was prolonged and intensive immersion in their societies. (Hart, 1999, p. 1)

Ethnography, uncertainty and the response to danger

The product of ethnographic fieldwork is a series of case studies of other cultures. As these cumulated during the 1920s and 1930s, it was clear that there were certain common themes, such as the importance of kinship relations for managing production and repro-duction in pre-modern societies and the key role of religious beliefs and activities in maintaining the order of the social and natural worlds. The issue of how these societies managed the intrinsic uncertainty of everyday life and sought to predict and manage the future was not one of these prominent themes. However, reading of classic anthropolo-gical texts indicates that they contain interesting insights that fit with some current themes in risk studies.

In the *Argonauts of the Western Pacific*, Malinowski explored the ways in which the Trobriand Islanders engaged in an inter-Island network of exchange, the Kula ring, involving dangerous long-distance sea voyages between Islands. This was a highly competitive enterprise in which the stakes were high; local leaders engaging in Kula exchange had to overcome obstacles and dangers and, if successful, increased their status and prestige. It was a form of voluntary risk taking (see Zinn, 2015).

Malinowski observed that the Islanders sought to mitigate the uncertainties and maximise the likelihood of success through a combination of technology and magic. For example, in building the large sea-going canoe used in the Kula trips, the owner of the canoe and his immediate relatives assemble the basic building block of the canoe, the main hollowed out tree trunk, planks, boards and role and the carved decorative prow boards. The owner then mobilised the community to assemble the canoe, build the outrigger and make the sail. This second stage was accompanied and punctuated by the performance of Kula magical rituals. Malinowski noted that the construction of canoes for the Kula exchange was 'permeated with tribal customs, ceremonial and magic, the last based on mythology' (Malinowski, 1999, p. 86).

In Malinowski's account, the two types of activity and the associated knowledge and skills were complementary. The technical and organisational boat building skills were based on instrumental rationality. He noted that:

> [Sea-going canoes] are …the greatest achievement of the craftsmanship of these natives… Technical difficulties face them, which require knowledge, and can only be overcome by a continuous, systematic effort and at certain stages must be met by means of communal labour. (Malinowski, 1999, pp. 86–87)

There was also an element of instrumental rationality in magic, for example, it contributed to the motivation and organisation of communal labour. However, it was essentially based on an act of faith (see Zinn's classification of responses to uncertainty 2008) about the successful outcome of the enterprise:

natives firmly believe in the value of magic… magic puts order and sequence into the various activities…it and its associated ceremonial are instrumental in securing the co-operation of the community, the organisation of community work… far from being a useless appendage, or even a burden on the work, supplies the psychological influence, which keeps the people confident about the success of their labour, and provides them with a natural leader [the magician]. (Malinowski, 1999, p. 88–89)

Malinowski argued that magic was based on the belief in supernatural 'superior power' that had 'the capacity to destroy human life and command other agents of destruction' but that 'magic also gives man the power and means to defend himself' (Malinowski, 1999, p. 393). Thus, for the Trobriand Islander, it 'is his weapon and armour against the many dangers which crowd in upon him on every side' (Malinowski, 1999, p. 393). Thus, in the Trobriand Islands, magic motivated the 'animal spirits', which the economist Keynes (1936, pp. 161–3) argued are needed when individuals have to make decisions and undertake activities under conditions of uncertainty, those in which they did not have the knowledge to calculate the likelihood of outcomes. As Zinn (2008) noted in late modern societies, there are equivalent strategies, such as hope, for enabling decision-making and actions when individuals are facing serious adversity. Rather than being part of shared collective experience and narratives as they are in the Trobriand Islands in late modern societies this response to uncertainty is grounded in individuals' biographies and experiences (see Alaszewski and Wilkinson's (2015) analysis of stroke survivors' response to the uncertainties of their everyday lives). They are enacted by the individual:

In everyday life [in late modern societies], there is rarely enough time and knowledge available for fully rational decision-making. Therefore, strategies such as trust, intuition, and emotions are of central importance to individuals' risk-balancing activities. (Zinn, 2008, 446)

Evans-Pritchard in his ethnographic study of the Azande published in 1937 as *Witchcraft, oracles and magic among the Azande* also addressed issues relating to the ways in which the Azande made decisions under conditions of uncertainty. He focused directly on how the Azande sought to predict and control the future, how they identified and accounted for misfortune, and how they allocated blame for such misfortune and sought to mitigate it.

Before any important undertaking, the Azande consulted one of their oracles to check that the outcome would be successful. The Azande had a range of oracles which they placed in order reliability; the rubbing board, termites and poison oracle (Evans-Pritchard, 1937, p. 353). The poison oracle had the highest status but was also the most expensive as it involved poisoning a chicken. The termite oracle involved no cost but took longer to make a prediction. It involved cutting the branches of two trees, inserting them into a termite hill and seeing whether the termites ate one or more branches overnight. The results had to be interpreted. If the question was whether misfortune would happen if a Zande decided to stay in his old homestead and both branches were eaten then the answer was yes and no which could be interpreted as 'the termites see good fortune in the immediate future but some misfortune a long way ahead' (Evans-Pritchard, 1937, p. 354). Evans-Pritchard observed that these oracles were central to the everyday life of the Azande and formed a crucial part of their decision-making:

If time and opportunity permitted many Azande would wish to consult one or other of the oracles about every step of their lives. (Evans-Pritchard, 1937, p. 264)

Evans-Pritchard noted that no Zande would undertake a major enterprise or expect another Zande to take part if he or she was unable to demonstrate a positive endorsement from an oracle. This is particularly evident in the case of large communal activities and in such circumstances the Azande consulted a witch doctor who could not only predict the future but could also take action to change it, for example, by counteracting hostile magical forces (Evans-Pritchard, 1937, p. 258). Thus, as with the magical ritual in the Trobriand Islands, the oracles converted future uncertainty about an enterprise into certainty enabling individuals and groups to act with confidence.

However, despite such precautions, individuals did experience misfortunes. Like the Trobriand Islanders, the Azande differentiated between the technical and magical or supernatural aspects of events. They recognised that the production of carved wooden bowls or clay pots depended on the quality of the material and the skill of the craftsmen but if a potter selected decent clay, made his pot properly and took precaution such as abstaining from sex on the night before he dug up the clay but a batch of pots broke when fired then there was an additional explanation, 'It is broken – there is witchcraft' (Evans-Pritchard, 1937, p. 67). Similarly, if a granary collapsed and killed the people sitting in its shade then:

> The Zande knows that the supports were undermined by termites and that people were sitting beneath the granary to escape the heat and glare of the sun. But he knows besides that these two events occurred at a precisely similar moment in time and space. It was due to the action of witchcraft (Evans-Pritchard, 1937, p. 70).

Thus, for Azande there are no accidents (see Green's (1999) analysis for the ways in which accident and chance are being eroded in late modern society). All aspects of misfortune could be explained; natural processes explained *how* they happened and witchcraft explained *why* specific individuals were harmed.

Douglas commented that witchcraft was part of everyday life amongst the Azande and they were adept at dealing with it. She commented that Evans-Pritchard felt that the Azande were amongst 'the most happy and carefree [people] of the Sudan' (Douglas, 1966, p. 1) and:

> The feelings of an Azande man, on finding he was bewitched, are not terror but hearty indignation as one of us might feel on finding himself the victim of embezzlement. (Douglas, 1966, p. 1)

Given the ubiquity of witchcraft, Evans-Pritchard examined the pattern of witchcraft accusations, who was accused of being a witch and blamed for an individual's misfortune. He found that witchcraft accusations followed and highlighted lines of internal social tension. Since witches attacked those they hated or were envious or jealous of:

> [a] Zande in misfortune at once considers who is likely to hate him. He is well aware that others take pleasure in his troubles and pain and are displeased at his good fortune. (Evans-Pritchard, 1937, p. 100)

For Evans-Pritchard, this pattern of accusation was one of the main functions of witchcraft amongst the Azande. It allowed social tensions to be articulated, made public and peacefully resolved. The relatives of the victim did not want to increase the anger of the witch, so they would make the accusation politely. The accused witch did not publically want to affirm that he intended to harm the victim, so he would undertake the ritual of blowing water on the wing of the bird killed by the poison oracle that had confirmed his witchcraft. This cooled his anger (Evans-Pritchard, 1937, pp. 97–98).

Evans-Pritchard's account of the Azande was a convincing analysis of the ways in which the Azande turned the potentially unmanageable uncertainty of everyday life into manageable certainty. Their various oracles enabled them to predict the future and identify and counteract danger. Witchcraft provided both an explanation and a mechanism for overtly dealing with misfortune and covertly with the underlying social tension and conflict. There were logical flaws in this the system. An epidemiologist would be puzzled by the Azande assertion that all deaths could be attributed to witchcraft but that counter magic was effective and killed the offending witch. However, Evans-Pritchard argued that the Azande did not reflect on the overall logic of their system, they were concerned about using it to deal with the practicalities of everyday life.

Beyond ethnographic case studies: accusations, pollution and danger

By the 1960s, the close relationship between social anthropology and ethnographic field-work was under pressure. Not only were other social science disciplines developing their own form of ethnography (for example Whyte an American sociologist in his study Italian slum in Boston originally published in 1943 (Whyte, 1993)) but some social anthropologists questioned the dominance of the ethnographic case study; in particular its failure to place the cultures and societies being studied into a broader temporal and social context. These anthropologists argued that for a fuller understanding of social change and inter-actions, anthropologists should not restrict themselves to ethnographic data but like Victorian armchair anthropologists should draw on a wide range of sources such as historical documents.

In France, this broader approach survived the move to ethnographic fieldwork. For example, leading members of the L'Année Sociologique used the techniques of armchair anthropology to great effect. Durkheim (1915) in *The Elementary Forms of Religious Life* first published in 1912 used a variety of sources including accounts of other cultures, especially those of Australian aboriginal cultures, as the basis of his theory of the development of religion in pre-modern societies. Mauss (2002) in the *The Gift*, first published in 1925, also used a variety of historic and ethnographic accounts, including Malinowski's study of the Kula ring. He reflected on the ways in which exchange and gift created mutual dependency, moral obligations and solidarity between social groups in pre-modern and archaic societies.

Lévi-Strauss, possibly the most influential twentieth century French anthropologist, built on this tradition. In the late 1930s, he was part of the French cultural mission to Brazil and with his wife he undertook some field trips into the Brazilian interior. Although these trips were short, weeks rather than the years of UK fieldworkers and he never learnt a native language or 'immersed' himself in a particular culture, his experiences shaped his subsequent career. Following a period of exile during the Second World War in the US, where he interacted with US anthropologists, he returned to France and was awarded his doctorate for an ethnographic study of Brazilian tribe and the accompanying theoretical analysis of kinship and marriage in pre-modern societies. This theoretical study was subsequently published in 1949 and its title, *The Elementary Structures of Kinship* (Lévi-Strauss, 1969), was a reference to Durkheim's classic, *The Elementary Forms of Religious Life*. Lévi-Strauss drew heavily on the Mauss' methods and theory. He admired Mauss' 'ability to assemble facts from entirely different times and places and compare them' (Lévi-Strauss in Massenzio, 2001, p. 423). Theoretically, Lévi-Strauss drew on Mauss' theory of exchange arguing that marriages in pre-modern societies formed part of systems of exchanges or alliances between social groups and that such exchanges were based on underlying structures of logic. This was a critique of the British anthropologists who saw marriage and kinship in functional terms and as descent from a common ancestor. Lévi-Strauss subsequently applied this structural approach to a major study of the myths of the Americas that rivalled Frazer's Golden Bough in scope and ambition; his science of mythology series eventually included four volumes that closely followed the approach he outlined in an early paper (Lévi-Strauss, 1955).

His aim in his study of mythology was to show how all myths in the Americas formed part of a single corpus and were based on logical transformations enabling Native Americans to address the basic questions of human existence. Like Fraser, he believed that modern science was superior to pre-modern magic, indeed this was one of the reasons why social systems based on scientific reasoning were replacing those based on magical reasoning and the urgency to record and understand systems based on magic. But, unlike Fraser he did not believe that magic was irrational, it was grounded in a different logic and rationality:

> I have to admit that scientific thought works and magical thought doesn't, that it was an attempt – actually, I am wrong in placing it in the past, because magic still exists and all of us are magical in one way or another... my objective in *The Savage Mind* [Lévi-Strauss, 1966] was... to place the thought of people without writing and that of so-called civilized people in some sort of equality, on the same plane... (Lévi-Strauss in Massenzio, 2001, p. 420)

While British anthropologists were interested in exploring the social functions of myths and magic, Lévi-Strauss was more interested in exploring the underlying logic, the system of symbols underpinning myth and magic. He wanted to use them as a way of gaining insight into the collective mental processes of pre-modern societies much as contemporary linguists were interested in the internal structure and logic of languages. Indeed, one of the reasons he shifted from a study of kinship to that of mythology was that mythology represented pure thought, unconstrained by the practicalities of kinship and marriage (Lévi-Strauss in Massenzio, 2001, p. 422). He used the watch analogy to describe his interest in myths noting that he was interested in the mechanisms or structures that caused the watch or myth to work – not the practical, personal and emotional consequences of measuring time or recounting myths (Lévi-Strauss in Massenzio, 2001, p. 421). His interest in the logical structure and links between myths did not stop him from reflecting on their meaning and accepting that they were reflections on the intrinsic mysteries or contradictions in human life. For example, he argued that the Oedipus myths addressed:

> the problem of understanding how one can be born from two: how is it that we do not have only one procreator but a mother plus a father? (Lévi-Strauss, 1955, p. 435).

In the UK, the post-war generation of anthropologists such as Leach and Douglas was moving in the same direction as Lévi-Strauss. For example, Leach, who had initially studied mathematics and engineering, applied his mathematic understanding of transfor-mations and his engineering understanding of structure. Leach noted that his analysis which he had completed in 1943 was recognised [by Lévi-Strauss] 'as having some kinship with his own work' (Leach, 1984, p. 17). In his post-war study of the Kachin of Highland Burma (Leach, 1954) based on fieldwork he started in 1939, Leach explicitly drew on Lévi-Strauss' analysis of kinship to explore the ways in which different patterns of marriage and exchange created different social and political formations (Leach, 1984, p. 18). Although Leach was disparaging of traditional ethnographic case studies, in which a 'cultural system [was described] as a unique self-sufficient, functioning whole' (Leach, 1984, p. 19), referring to this as 'butterfly collecting' (Leach, 1984, p. 19), he did considered that he remained a British 'empiricist' as, unlike Lévi-Strauss, he was unwilling to make the facts fit the theory.

Douglas, like Lévi-Strauss, was willing to use a wide range of sources both historical and contemporary and was interested in the logic underpinning human action. In the late 1930s and 1940s, she studied in Oxford with Evans-Pritchard undertaking fieldwork with the Lele in the Belgian Congo which formed the basis of an ethnographic study (Douglas, 1963). Douglas did not see Lele as a static stable society, for example, she devoted a chapter to the impact of Europeans on the Lele. She also noted that responses to sorcery accusations had changed, for example, the Belgians had outlawed poison oracles and there were messianic anti-sorcery cults that periodically swept through Lele villages. As in Evans-Pritchard's study of the Azande, Douglas noted that there was a pattern to accusations, but in contrast to the witchcraft accusations amongst the Azande which followed lines of tensions within local communities, Lele sorcery accusations focussed on breaches of ritual purity and on outsiders; the dead, sorcerers in other villages and those who had left the village.

Douglas used these insights to develop a theoretical understanding of witchcraft in pre-modern cultures in Africa and in other cultures including European. There were two important and linked dimensions to this theorising; the symbolism of witchcraft and how its dangers were articulated and the relationship between patterns of accusations and different social structures.

Douglas argued that witchcraft was grounded in a series of binary symbols; active/passive, aggressive/vulnerable, inside/outside, good/bad and pure/contaminated or polluted. She noted that:

> The witch is an attacker and deceiver. He uses what is impure and potent to harm what is pure and helpless. The symbols what we recognise across the globe as witchcraft all build on the theme of vulnerable internal goodness attacked by external power. (Douglas, 1970, p. xxvi)

For example, she included in her edited collection on witchcraft, Forge's analysis of witchcraft amongst the Abelam, a tribe who live in the Sepik area of New Guinea. The witch is a local rival who steals bodily, especially sexual excretions from an individual, and pays a foreign sorcerer to mix it with magic paint to bewitch and kill the victim (Forge, 1970, p. 263). As Douglas noted this is an excellent example of witchcraft symbolism; contaminating material to make 'a... conscious attack from the outside upon the unconscious, unsuspecting, interior self' (Douglas, 1970).

Douglas (1970, pp. xxiv–xxxv) also noted that the existence of witchcraft and the pattern of witchcraft accusations reflected specific social settings. She noted that:

> Where social interactions are intense and ill defined, there may we expect to find witchcraft belief. Where human relations are sparse or diffuse, or where roles are fully ascribed, we do not expect to find witchcraft belief. (Douglas, 1970, p. xxxv)

Douglas cited Lienhardt's (1970) comparison of Nuer-Dinka (in Southern Sudan) with the closely related Anuak (1970, p. 279). The Nuer-Dinka followed their cattle and therefore lived far more solitary lives than the Anuak so that 'Anuak are interested in people, Dinka-Nuer are more interested in cattle' (Lienhardt, 1970, p. 279). The intense politicking of Anuak village life was associated with intense interest in death and its human causes such as sorcery and curses. In contrast, the Nuer-Dinka showed little interest in human intrigue, witchcraft and death. Instead they concentrated on placating the Deity that controlled the pastures they and their cattle depended on.

Douglas argued that the specific arrangement of witchcraft symbols depended on the nature of the social setting:

> the way in which the witch works, his sources of power, the nature of his attack on his victim all these can be related to an image of the community and the kind of attack to which the community values are subject. (Douglas, 1970, p. xxviii)

Douglas elaborated these ideas considering them in contexts outside witchcraft and developing important insights into the social structuring of the perceptions and management of risk. In *Purity and Danger* (Douglas, 1966, 2002), she developed her theoretical insight into the symbolic systems that underpin the articulation of threats, dangers or risk to specific social groups.

While Douglas noted that witchcraft was restricted to specific social settings, she argued in *Purity and Danger* (Douglas, 1966) that one of the key elements of witchcraft, the symbolic binary purity/impurity division and the associated process of contamination resulting from the mixing of the pure and impure are important in both pre-modern and modern societies. This division has important social functions; purity is essentially benign and shapes cultural definitions of order, normality and safety whereas impurity is powerful but dangerous and underpins cultural definitions of disorder, abnormality and otherness. Thus, purity and impurity shape the ways in which social groups account for past misfortunes and how they identify and seek to manage future threats.

In *Purity and Danger*, Douglas (1966) explored the ways in which definitions of purity were grounded in systems of logic and reason that were embedded in different social systems and cultures. For example, dirt, a form of impurity, is essentially matter out of place; soil on a field is in the right place but in a 'clean' house it is dirt. Douglas, like Lévi-Strauss, was interested in such symbolic systems of classification as they offered insight into the ways in which different communities reflected on the fundamental issues of human existence:

> Reflection on dirt involves reflection on the relation of order to disorder, being to non-being, form to formlessness, life to death. Wherever ideas of dirt are highly structured their analysis disclose a play on such profound themes. (Douglas, 1966, p. 5)

Douglas noted that each social group had its own logical system that provided a classification of nature and its relationship to man. Contemporary anthropologists were also researching issues of ethnobotany. For example, Bulmer (1967) examined why the Karam people living in highland New Guinea who 'show an enormous, detailed and on the whole highly accurate knowledge of natural history' did not classify the Cassowary as a bird or group dogs with other animals. He concluded that both animals defied classification as they enjoyed a 'unique relationship in Karam thought to man' (Bulmer, 1967, p. 5). He also noted how taxonomy was linked to edibility of different types of animals:

> Thus Karam explain that they do not eat 'rats' (kopyak), certain small birds, and indeed almost any other creatures found around the homesteads except the domestic pig, on the grounds that these eat or are otherwise associated with excrement, unclean foods and female dirt, and with the corpses which are exposed in open, fenced graves near the houses in the first stage of the disposal of the dead. (Bulmer, 1967, p. 9)

Douglas also reflected on the ways in which some animals defied classification. For example, in her fieldwork amongst the Lele, Douglas (1963) identified the anomalous and unique position of the pangolin. The pangolin did not fit Lele taxonomy of animals: it was a forest animal but had scales like fish, unlike other animals it did not produce multiple offspring and when threatened by hunters did not run away but rolled into a ball. The Lele considered the pangolin to be unclean and highly dangerous to eat but it was the centre of Lele ritual. A key part of these rituals involved killing and eating the pangolin. Douglas saw this was a way in which the Lele addressed the basic contradictions of their existence:

> The inner cult of all their ritual life, in which the initiates of the pangolin, immune to the dangers that would kill uninitiated men, approach, hold and kill and eat the animal which in its own existence combines all the features which Lele culture keeps apart... They [Lele] dare to grasp the pangolin and put it to ritual use, proclaiming this has more power than any other rites. So the pangolin cult is capable of inspiring profound meditation on the nature of purity and impurity and on the limitations on human contemplation of existence.
>
> Not only does the pangolin overcome the distinctions in the universe. Its power for good is released by its dying and this it seems to take on itself deliberately (Douglas, 1966, p. 170).

Douglas (1966, pp. 41–57) applied the same approach to historical sources most notably the animal taxonomy and associated classification as animals as unclean abominations the Old Testament of the Bible (Deuteronomy and Leviticus) such as camels and pigs. Douglas argued that animals were considered to be unclean and therefore inedible if they confounded the underlying logic of animal classification. In this taxonomy, clean edible animals chewed the cud and had clove hoofs. Camels and pigs were unclean as they breached these taxonomic rules; camels chewed the cud but did not have cloven hoofs while pigs had cloven hoofs but did not chew the cud (Douglas, 1966, pp. 41–42). Douglas rejected the various explanations of these dietary rules including proto-scientific or medical explanations that the ban was a hygiene measure to prevent spread of disease from dirty scavenging pigs to humans. She emphasised the ways in which adherence to these rules made mundane actions such as preparing food into symbolic statements about the membership of a religious community.

There was criticism of Douglas' analyses from some social anthropologists. For example, Bulmer felt that her analysis of the pangolin cult was firmly anchored in ethnographic research but her analysis of Biblical sources was not. He argued that there was not enough ethnographic data to provide the full context for the biblical taxonomies and associated classification. For example, he noted that pigs might be placed in a special taxonomic category because eating them was considered to be dangerous to human health rather than their inedibility stemming from their anomalous taxonomic status (Bulmer, 1967, p. 21). Furthermore, the ancient Israelites could be using the ban of pig eating to differentiate themselves and their god from 'pig-eating' neighbouring peoples and their gods. In her preface to the 2002 edition of *Purity and Danger*, Douglas acknowledged the criticism and shifted the emphasis of her analysis from the uncleanness, inedibility and abnormality of pigs and camels to the cleanness, edibility and sacredness of cattle and sheep. She argued that as pastoralists the ancient Israelites were dependent on the wellbeing of their cattle and sheep and to ensure this they ritually killed and sacrificed cows and sheep to their God. Thus, each meal in which they killed and ate a cow or sheep was symbolically linked to their covenant with both their herds and God and so that: 'The dietary laws intrinsically model the body and altar on each other' (Douglas, 2002, p. xvi).

In her work, Douglas highlighted a number of major themes that are central to the study of risk:

- *The difference between danger and risk.* She noted that all social groups have to deal with a range of social and natural hazards or dangers. However, constraints of time and resources mean individuals can only worry about some of these and these become risks. The selection of risks reflects social and political relations within groups.

  'Dangers are manifold and omnipresent. Action would be paralysed if individuals attended to all of them; anxiety has to be selective. We draw on the idea that risk is like taboo. Arguments about risk are highly charged, morally and politically. Naming a risk amounts to an accusation' (Douglas, 2002, p. xix).
- *Boundaries are critical to the identification of risk.* There are some boundaries that are important in most societies, for example, the boundaries of the body and the boundary of the social group and these two boundaries are often symbolically linked.

  'We cannot possibly interpret rituals concerning excreta, breast milk, saliva and the rest unless we are prepared to see in the body a symbol of society, and to see the powers and dangers credited to social structures reproduced in small on the human body' (Douglas, 1966, p. 115).

  These boundaries are protected by physical and magical means, such as taboos. For example, in some societies those accused of breaching moral boundaries were physically disfigured, stigmatised, whereas in others those tasked with maintaining these boundaries had to be unblemished. For example, Leviticus specifies that a priest 'must be a perfect man' (Douglas, 1966, p. 51).
- *Crossing boundaries is risky and may require special ritual action to ensure protection.* Douglas drew on Van Gennep's (2010) classic study of rites of passage originally published in 1909 noting that Van Gennep

  'saw society as house with rooms and corridors in which the passage from one to another is dangerous. Danger lies in the transitional states, simply because transition is neither one state nor the next, it is undefinable. The person who must pass from one to another is himself in danger and emanated danger to others. The danger is controlled by ritual...' (Douglas, 1966, p. 96).
- *Otherness: insiders and outsider.* Douglas (1966, pp, 94–113) noted that social groups seek to maintain internal order while resisting external threats and therefore the symbolic structuring and boundary between inside and outside are important Within the boundaries of a social group, outsiders, individuals who did not conform to established custom and practices, presented a potential threat to order because of their abnormality or otherness. For example, she described the roots of anti-Semitism and the anomalous position of Jews in the English society in the following way:

  'Belief in their sinister but undeniable advantages in commerce justifies discrimination against them – whereas their real offence is always to be outside the formal structure of Christendom' (Douglas, 1966, p. 104).
- *The social structuring of risk and perceptions of danger.* In *Purity and Danger*, Douglas (1966) noted the ways in which the intensity and competiveness of social

relations shaped perceptions of dangers such as witchcraft. In a later work, Douglas (2003) proposed a typology of the social structure based on individual's strength of allegiance to a social group (grid) and the control which the group exerted over the individual (group). Douglas argued that these two factors shape the ways in which individuals perceived risk and responded to danger. For example, groups that are high-group and are grounded in strong control of individuals tend to 'expel and downgrade dissenters' (Douglas, 2003, p. 6).

Comment: Douglas' work is important for risk studies. She provides a major point of contact between the ethnographic research and risk studies. Her interest in risk and danger grew out of her initial ethnographic work on the Lele, albeit unlike many contemporary anthropologists her ethnography grounded the Lele in real time and space exploring issues of interaction with other social groups and processes of social change. The Lele provided a rich source of data on risk issues in terms of their taxonomies of the natural world including anomalies such as the pangolin, their concern with maintaining purity and the role of rituals in maintaining purity and order through testing boundaries, for example, in the pangolin cult and their anxieties about the internal threat of sorcery. In *Purity and Danger*, Douglas (1966) was able to build on this work by drawing on a wider range of historical and contemporary evidence. She convincingly argued that risk cannot not be reduced to objective deficits in the natural world or to processes of individual psychology. Indeed, risk logics are shaped by symbolic systems expressed in various systems of classifications and taxonomies. Those who use these systems take them for granted and therefore the underlying symbolism can only be identified through systematic ethnographic study of risk perceptions. She adopted a 'soft constructionist' approach (Lupton, 1999) noting that real dangers do exist but that only some of these became risks and the process of selection, risk perception, is socially structured. Real misfortunes happen, people fall ill and become sick, even die, but the response to such misfortune, the pattern of accusations, the identification of who is to be blamed, is socially and politically structured. The term witch hunt may be used metaphorically in modern societies but it is shaped by the same social processes that underpin witch hunts in pre-modern communities.

However, there are limitations to Douglas' analyses of risk and danger. Like other theoretical accounts grounded in ethnographic data, the emphasis tends to be on the underlying social processes and symbolism rather than on the active role of the individual. For example, ethnographic case studies such as Malinowski's account of kula exchange emphasise the nature of uncertainty for individual participants; the Trobriand islanders planning their kula trip have to deal with many uncertainties both about the journey and about the exchange itself. However, in theoretical accounts of such exchanges by Mauss and Lévi-Strauss the active role of the individual in managing uncertainty is lost and the emphasis is on the structure of exchange. As Bourdieu observed in these theories of exchange:

> the 'automatic laws' of the cycle of reciprocity are the unconscious principle of the obligation to give, the obligation to return a gift and the obligation to receive... the analyst reduces agents to status of automata... uncertainly remains the outcome of the interaction until the whole cycle is complete. The most ordinary and even the most seemingly routine exchanges of ordinary life, like the 'little gifts' that 'bind friendship', presuppose an improvisation, and therefore a constant uncertainty, which, makes all their charm, and hence all their social efficiency. (1990, pp. 98–99)

In this observation, Bourdieu highlights the key role of time. Individuals living their everyday life do so within time; they make sense and account for past misfortunes and plan their future activities. Researchers observing these activities can and often do extract them from time; with the benefit of hindsight, the focus is on the predictability rather than uncertainty of exchanges.

Developing the relationship between anthropology and risk studies

The relationship between anthropology and risk has been fruitful. A rereading from a risk perspective of classic texts and Douglas' analyses generate insights into the relationship between health, risk and society. However, there is scope for developing the relationship in terms of subject matter and in terms of exploring the co-existence of different ways of managing uncertainty. There was, in twentieth century social science, a residue of nineteenth century evolutionary theorising, particularly in the assertion that western science and technology provided superior access to the truth than other culture's religion and magic and through globalisation would replace them. However there is evidence that both religion and magic are resilient and remain important in all societies. Such resilience means that anthropologists should reflect on how these different responses coexist and how and when they are used to manage uncertainty.

Typologies of societies: magic, religion and science

In both anthropology and sociology, there has been a tendency to consider modern and pre-modern societies in binary terms. In social science, pre-modern societies tend to be characterised as small scale, rural and based on face-to-face relations, dominated by localised subsistence production and exchange, with oral transmission of knowledge, a key element of this knowledge is religious belief and practices. In social science accounts, such societies are represented as essentially unchanging and homeostatic.

In contrast, modern societies are characterised as large-scale, urban with networks of relations maintained over time and space through various forms of communication, production and exchange that generate surpluses of sophisticated goods and are globalised and based on a complex division of labour linked to systematic creation and storage of essentially secular scientific knowledge in various forms of written texts. Such societies are seen as constantly changing and developing.

These differences can be linked to differences in ways in which risk is articulated and managed. In small-scale pre-modern societies, magic and supernatural forces play a key role; they explain individual and collective misfortune, provide the basis for divination enabling the prediction of the future and are the key resource which experts use to identify and counter hostile forces. In modern societies, scientific knowledge provides the key resource which experts such as doctors use to explain misfortune and use to identify and counter threats such as serious illness. MacFarlane in a discussion of the use of witchcraft as an explanation of personal misfortune noted that:

> In a small-scale, 'face-to-face' society where there are few specialized relationships and where close personal bonds serve most men's interests 'all events tend to be explained by what occurs in those relationships' [and personal ill-will] (MacFarlane, 1999, p. 194).

However, it is possible to identify societies that share characteristics of both types. Such historic societies or civilisations such as classic Greece, Rome, China or Japan were based on small scale subsistence production and exchanges that generated a surplus that supported more sophisticated urban centres that could be substantial and include major complex systems of production and division of labour. Most of the communication in these societies was small-scale, face-to-face and most communication was oral but there existed alongside this more sophisticated systems based on the production and storage of texts both religious and secular which could form the basis of creation, storage and instruction in the knowledge contained in these texts.

The study of such societies has been led by archaeologists and historians who focus on the texts and artefacts which have survived that provide accounts of activities of supernatural being such as gods and their interaction with humans and sites of ritual practices to influence the behaviour of these gods. There are also texts that indicate how individuals sought to engage supernatural forces in their everyday life. As Brown (1970) observed in the study of late Roman antiquity (200–600 CE) magical papyri and lead cursing-tablets provide an insight into the technology of witchcraft and sorcery but provide less information on the social dynamics of accusations (Brown, 1970, pp. 18–19). He showed that in the fourth century both pagan and Christians believed that 'demons were the effective agents of all misfortune' (Brown, 1970, pp. 28) though their actions were influenced by human agents, sorcerers who controlled demons and cursers who exposed those they cursed to demons. By the sixth century, the Christianisation of the Empire meant that the agents were outsiders, witches who entered a compact with the devil or Jews who denied Christ (Brown, 1970. p. 35). By examining accounts of the elite, Brown was able to place hostile magical attacks within their social context. He argued that 'points of uncertainty and conflict in the social structure of the governing classes of the Empire' (Brown, 1970. p. 21) were linked to the ways in which members of the elite explained their personal misfortunes as caused insiders by 'pinning the blame on individuals' (Brown, 1970. p.19). In contrast, public and collective misfortune was directed at outsiders and explained:

> in this age of bitter confessional hatreds, by the anger of the gods or God at the existence of dissenting religious groups – Christians, pagans, or heretics. (Brown, 1970, p. 19)

Similarly, Macfarlane (1999) drew on anthropological theory and documentary sources to examine the rise and fall of witchcraft accusations in sixteenth and seventeenth century England, especially in the County of Essex. He showed that the accusations rose rapidly in the fifteenth and sixteenth century and then declined, disappearing by the eighteenth century. There was a clear pattern to the accusations, more affluent farmers tended to accuse their poorer female neighbours of causing misfortune in their family. MacFarlane argued the pattern of accusations was related to both religious and social changes. He suggested that Pre-Reformation Catholicism provided both an explanation and a way of responding to misfortune without 'the blame being centred on either the individual or his neighbours' (Macfarlane 1999, p. 195). Following the reformation Puritan writers noted the 'connexion between sin and disease, or between suffering and human failure' (Macfarlane 1999, p. 194). In principle, blame could be allocated to the individual's own moral failing, to the evil or malice of neighbours or to God testing the individual. The Puritans focussed on the first and the third cause, those making witchcraft accusations highlighted the malice of neighbours. Macfarlane argued that the rise of accusations reflected social change including great disparity of wealth inside village communities and the decline in traditional mutual support and almsgiving prior to the development of more systematic systems of support such as the poor laws. Thus, witchcraft accusation formed part of the transition from pre-modern to modern society:

> Witchcraft beliefs can be seen as a form of reciprocal relationship. One neighbour injures another, both on the physical level, by refusing a gift, but also, more generally, by denying the existence of the mutual relationship. The witch reciprocates on two levels also, through a physical attack which is accompanied by a malice equivalent to that of the victim (Macfarlane 1999, p. 197).

While such historical accounts provide interesting insights, they tend to be restricted to European history. There is scope for applying the same approach to other complex pre-modern societies that have rich documentary sources such as Japan.

Globalisation: the end of magic and religion?

There is an assumption that given the superiority of technical, scientific and organisational systems of modern society, pre-modern societies will be absorbed into a single globalised social system. Sociologists, Albrow and King, defined globalisation as: 'all those pro-cesses by which the peoples of the world are incorporated into a single world society' (1990, p. 8). This process of globalisation involves the destruction traditional systems of dealing with misfortune based on magic and religion and their replacement with modern systems based on science, such as medicine. However, I shall argue that both magic and religions remain important in modern societies and that one important issue is how magic, religion and science interact and are used.

As I have noted the pioneering work of the 1898 Torres Island Strait Expedition was motivated by a desire to record the traditional culture and lives of islanders before they were irrevocably changed by their contact with western societies (Herle & Rouse, 1998). Lévi-Strauss saw the role of anthropologists as recording disappearing societies:

> A past extending back centuries and millennia and hundreds of millennia to the time when humankind began has presented us with small societies that were to become very numerous, each of which gave rise to original ways of life, irreplaceable beliefs, forms of oral or pictorial or sculptural expression constituting something unique in human experience and my role as an ethnographer was, to the extent that these have survived until the past one or two centuries and we can approach them through texts and objects and direct experience in fieldwork, to preserve something of this richness and diversity so that humankind in other forms, forms absolutely different from those that existed in the past, will be acquainted with them. (Lévi-Strauss in Massenzio, 2001, p. 42)

Anthropologists tended to see pre-modern societies as unchanging and unchangeable with no independent future. Although fieldworkers in the first part of the twentieth century worked in the context of colonialism, they tended to bracket this out in their ethnogra-phies. For example, Malinowski noted that his fieldwork took place on the Pacific Island that had:

> the products of the Standard Oil Company... [and] the ubiquitous motor launch. I was still able with little effort to re-live and reconstruct a type of human life moulded by the implements of the stone age, pervaded with crude beliefs and surrounded by a wide, uncontaminated open stretch of nature. (Malinowski quoted in Young, 1979, p. 16)

However, these societies have not been unchanging and make their own adjustments to new contacts. Modern systems penetrated such societies but often co-exist with the existing systems creating parallel systems which individuals can and do move between. This can be most clearly seen in the area of magic and religion. Commentators on globalisation have tended to accept the nineteenth century evolutionary assumption that scientific knowledge and institutions will replace those based on magic and religion. In the early 2000s, it is clear that both religion and magic are resilient as are pre-modern societies, even in those areas of modern life, which are grounded in risk rationality such as modern medicine.

Survival and adaptation: there is evidence that the defining features of some pre-modern societies which anthropologists observed and recorded in the early twentieth century remain important in the late twentieth and early twenty-first centuries. As Young noted in his edited collection of Malinowski's ethnography: the Kula... continues to operate within and between the Trobriand Islands and Dobu, though in a somewhat modified form (Young, 1979, p. 20). A documentary broadcast on British Broadcasting Corporation (BBC; 10 May 2015, Hunters of the South Pacific: The Kula Ring) made it clear that there had been substantial changes on the Island with the development of mass tourism and a money economy. This undermined large scale Kula expeditions as Islanders could earn money from tourism and spend it in local shops. The documentary showed how Kula and the high status shell armband and necklaces remained valuable items and an important resource for individuals wanting to maintain their traditional status and way of life.

It is also evident that amongst the Azande oracles and witchcraft remain an important part of everyday life. When Jonathan Miller, a qualified doctor, actor and producer visited Zandeland in 1976 to research and film the Azande for his BBC documentary, *The Body in Question* (Miller, 1978), he found that 'belief in the existence of witches persists' (Miller, 1978, p. 87) and that it continued to be an explanation for all misfortune:

> When someone falls ill in Zandeland, he does not suspect witchcraft in general; he attributes his illness to witchcraft or sorcery of particular people with whom he has already has a quarrel. In other words, the diagnostic techniques employed by the Azande articulate pre-existing grudges and grievances (Miller 1978, p. 89)

In a documentary entitled *Witchcraft amongst the Azande* in the Granada anthropology series 'Disappearing World' first broadcast in 1982, it was clear that rural Zandeland had been penetrated by the institutions of western culture. Local villagers attended church and justice was dispensed by the police and the magistrate, a local chief, all dressed in western-style uniforms. However, it quickly became clear in the documentary that the changes were relatively superficial. For example, the magistrate used the poison oracle to decide the facts in an adultery accusation case. Fifty years after Evans-Pritchard's field-work, the documentary recorded the same response to misfortune, witchcraft, the use of the same oracles, termites, rubbing board and poison oracles and the use of witch doctors and magic to neutralise threat and danger.

Managing the relationship between traditional life and modern systems: given that traditional ways of life and systems of understanding and managing the world are often resilient, one issue relates to how traditional and modern systems coexist and interact and how individuals reconcile them. Gjernes (2008) explored this issue by examining how Sámi women, an ethnic minority in Northern Norway who maintain a traditional reindeer herding life style, responded to expert advice grounded in rational risk assessment – whereby environmental experts advised them to move away from reindeer herding and medical experts advised them to adopt a more healthy life style. Gjernes noted that Sámi women rejected the environmental message as they were committed to the preservation of their culture and way of life:

> The women state that they try to socialise their children into Sámi ethnicity and the reindeer herding culture: it is part of their role to communicate the value of the herding business as a way of life and make sure the next generation gets the knowledge necessary to be in the business and to practice their culture (Gjernes, 2008, pp. 508–509).

Sámi women were aware of and understood the health promotion messages and wanted to show that they were responsible people, in touch with and responsive to the external world (Gjernes, 2008, p. 514). However, they interpreted these messages within their cultural context and value systems. For example, they interpreted expert advice to reduce their consumption of fatty food as advice to continue eating healthy, natural lean reindeer meat but not to eat unhealthy artificially produced fatty lamb. Gjernes noted that:

> Reindeer herding is meat production, and the reindeer herders eat what they produce. For these respondents, to consume meat indicates relative wealth and high protein content makes meat a valuable source of food… [as one respondent stated]
>
> *I believe reindeer meat is very healthy, because it is lean, you know that lamb is very fat and we hardly eat it at all. The animals are living outdoors, eating natural food like reindeer moss and hay. But we also eat food made of blood, we make sausages from it, and I consider that to be a very healthy food.*
>
> …. Here, 'natural' may be seen to represent 'purity,' which the respondents also seem to consider as less risky than modern 'industrially' produced meat (Gjernes, 2008, p. 509).

For these Sámi women, life style, cultural identity and risk were interconnected. Health risk was not a separate distinctive category of danger. As Gjernes argued: 'the women's accounts refer to more than a health discourse; it is also a cultural discourse connected to positive aspects of ethnicity, food habits and the general advantages of consuming reindeer meat' (2008, 509).

Magic in modern systems: the existence of magic in modern societies is not just a phenomenon related to the survival of pre-modern belief and practices. Modern systems grounded in scientific knowledge can and do contain magical elements. The American sociologist, Roth (1957), undertook a study of hospitals treating patients with tuberculosis. Roth observed that the hospital undertook measures to minimise the risk of infection. Senior hospital staff claimed that these measures were based on rational risk management, but given the uncertainty about nature of the dangers and failure to apply these measures consistently such measures were magical:

> These uncertainties [about infectiousness] leave the way open for ritualized procedures that often depend more on convenience and ease of administration than on rationally deduced probabilities. They also leave the way open for irrational practices that can properly be called 'magic.' (Roth, 1957, p. 310)

Roth reached this conclusion by examining the ways in which protective devices such as masks, gloves and gowns were used. He found that their use was shaped by social not biological factors including: power, the most powerful groups doctors tended to avoid such protection; spatial factors, interactions in non-clinical spaces tended not to included protective barriers; and temporal, the 'rules suggest that the tubercle bacillus works only during business hours' (Roth, 1957, p. 313–4).

Globalisation and the continuing importance of belief in supernatural powers: Turner, in his analysis of globalisation, argued that religion and the belief in the influence of supernatural power on human activity, remains a potent force in the modern world. He identified historical continuities in interpretations of the causes of major collective disasters or misfortune:

> In the past, catastrophes such as the Black Death, the fire of London and the Lisbon earthquake produced major religious responses... The Asian tsunami resulted in a powerful religious response in fundamentalist circles in Indonesia, where video-tapes were soon available showing that the natural disaster was a punishment from God for human wickedness in Thailand and elsewhere (Turner, 2007, p. 689).

Turner noted that globalisation and the associated movement of people produced new forms of religion including hybrid religions and fundamentalism. He argued that new 'hybrid forms of religion are often constructed self-consciously and they are closely related to youth movements and to generational politics' (Turner, 2007, p. 679), while fundamentalists seek a purified version of religion. Turner observed that fundamentalism should not be equated with traditionalist retreat from the modern world as fundamentalist engaged with modern technologies such as social media. However it was a conscious rejection of the contamination of cultural hybridisation:

> There is obviously evidence to show how fundamentalism has attempted to contain the growth of cultural hybridization, to preserve what is seen to be the pristine, authentic faith, to sustain religious authority and orthodoxy, and in particular to curb the growth of women's social and political autonomy (Turner, 2007, p. 679).

Comment: while there is clearly an interaction between cultures, it does not seem that is a simple case of the dominant western culture absorbing all other cultures. In some situations pre-modern cultures continue to function albeit under a veneer of western practice, in other situations there is a process of hybridisation where elements of different cultures merge together but in other situations there may be a deliberate rejection of western culture and its institutions and a deliberate 'return' to the fundamentals of a religious system. These different responses involve different ways of constructing and managing uncertainty. How and why individuals and groups develop or adopt different responses is not understood and requires more study.

Conclusion

Anthropology especially in the United Kingdom has been a very distinctive and separate social science discipline, with its own methods, ethnographic fieldwork, and its own subject matter, small-scale oral pre-modern societies. While risk and uncertainty have not been central themes, ethnographic case studies such as Malinowski's studies of the Trobriand Island, Evans-Pritchard studies of the Azande and Douglas' studies of the Lele have generated important insights into the ways in which these societies account for the misfortunes and use divination and magic to manage the uncertainties of everyday life. Douglas' later work syntheses a range of evidence to examine these processes across time and between different social groups.

While the rise of science and the development of rational risk analysis seem to create risk technologies that provide the objective basis for identifying the causes of disasters and misfortunes and for avoiding them, such technologies have intrinsic limitations. Unlike Azande witchcraft they cannot explain why a particular individual suffered a particular misfortune at a particular moment of time. Nor can they change uncertainty into absolute certainty in the same way as magic; probability reduces but does not eliminate uncertainty. The optimism of eighteenth century enlightenment thinkers and nineteenth century anthropologists that scientific rationality would replace magical and religious (ir)rationality now seems misplaced. The question is not how science replaces magic and religion but how they coexist and relate to each other and how and in what circumstances individuals, groups and organisations use each.

Disclosure statement

No potential conflict of interest was reported by the author.

References

Alaszewski, A., & Wilkinson, I. (2015). The paradox of hope for working age adults recovering from stroke. *Health*, *19*(2), 172–187.

Albrow, M., & King, E. (Eds.). (1990). *Globalization, knowledge and society*. London: Sage.

Beattie, J. (1964). *Other cultures: Aims, methods and achievements in social anthropology*. London: Cohen & West.

Bourdieu, P. (1990). *The logic of practice*. Cambridge: Polity in association with Blackwell.

Brown, P. (1970). Sorcery, demons, and the rise of Christianity from late Antiquity into the Middle Ages. In M. Douglas (Ed.), *Witchcaft, confessions and accusations* (pp. 17–46). ASA Monographs 9. London: Tavistock Publications.

Bulmer, R. (1967). Why is the cassowary not a bird? A problem of zoological taxonomy among the Karam of the New Guinea highlands. *Man*, New Series *2*(1), 5–25. doi:10.2307/2798651

Caesar, J. (1996). *Seven commentaries on the Gallic Wars*. (C. Hammond, Trans.). Oxford: Oxford University Press.

Douglas, M. (1963). *The Lele of Kasai*. Oxford: Oxford University Press.

Douglas, M. (1966). *Purity and danger: An analysis of concept of pollution and taboo*. London: Routledge and Kegan Paul.

Douglas, M. (1970). Introduction: Thirty years after witchcraft, oracles and magic. In M. Douglas (Ed.), *Witchcaft, confessions and accusations* (pp. xiii–xxxviii). ASA Monographs 9. London: Tavistock Publications.

Douglas, M. (2002). *Purity and Danger: An analysis of concept of pollution and taboo*. (Routledge Classic Edition). London: Routledge.

Douglas, M. (2003). Introduction to grid/group analysis. In M. Douglas (Eds), *Essays in the sociology of perception: Collected works* (Vol. *VIII*, pp. 1–8). Abingdon, Oxon: Routledge.

Durkheim, E. (1915). *The elementary forms of the religious life*. (J.W. Swain, Trans.). London: G. Allen & Unwin.

Evans-Pritchard, E. E. (1937). *Witchcraft, oracles and magic among the Azande*. Oxford: The Clarendon Press.

Forge, A. (1970). Prestige, influence, and sorcery: A new guinea example. In M. Douglas (Ed.), *Witchcaft, confessions and accusations* (pp. 257–275). ASA Monographs 9. London: Tavistock Publications.

Frazer, S. (n.d.). *The golden bough: A study of magic and religion*. Retrieved April 21, 2015, from http://www.gutenberg.org/files/3623/3623-h/3623-h.htm

Gjernes, T. (2008). Perceptions of risk and uncertainty among Sámi women involved in reindeer herding in Northern Norway. *Health, Risk & Society*, *10*(5), 505–516. doi:10.1080/13698570802381154

Green, J. (1999). From accidents to risk: Public health and preventable injury. *Health, Risk & Society*, *1*(1), 25–39. doi:10.1080/13698579908407005

Hart, K. (1999). The Cambridge Torres Strait expedition and British social anthropology. *Memory Bank*. Retrieved from http://thememorybank.co.uk/2009/11/06/the-cambridge-torres-strait-expedition-and-british-social-anthropology/

Herle, A., & Rouse, S. (Eds.). (1998). *Cambridge and the torres strait: Centenary essays on the 1898 anthropological expedition*. Cambridge: Cambridge University Press.

Keynes, J. M. (1936). *A general theory of employment, interest and money*. London: Macmillan.

Leach, E. R. (1954). *Political systems of highland Burma: A study of Kachin structure*. London: Bell for the London School of Economics.

Leach, E. R. (1984). Glimpses of the unmentionable in the history of British social anthropology. *Annual Review of Anthropology, 13*, 1–24. doi:10.1146/annurev.an.13.100184.000245

Lévi-Strauss, C. (1955). The structural study of Myth. *The Journal of American Folklore, 68*(270), 428–444. doi:10.2307/536768

Lévi-Strauss, C. (1966). *The savage mind*. Chicago: University of Chicago Press.

Lévi-Strauss, C. (1969). *The elementary structures of kinship* (revised ed.). Boston, MA: Beacon Press.

Lienhardt, G. (1970). The situation of death: An aspect of Anuak philosophy. In M. Douglas (Ed.), *Witchcaft, confessions and accusations* (pp. 279–291). ASA Monographs 9. London: Tavistock Publications.

Lupton, D. (1999). *Risk*. London: Routledge.

Macfarlane, A. (1999). *Witchcraft in Tudor and Stuart England: A regional and comparative study* (2nd ed.). London: Routledge.

Malinowski, B. (1999). *Argonauts of the Western Pacific*. London: Routledge.

Massenzio, M. (2001). An interview with Claude Levi-Strauss. *Current Anthropology, 42*(3), 419–425. doi:10.1086/ca.2001.42.issue-3

Mauss, M. (2002). *The gift: The form and reason for exchange in archaic societies*. London: Routledge.

Miller, J. (1978). *The body in question*. London: Jonathan Cape.

Roth, J. A. (1957). Ritual and magic in the control of contagion. *American Sociological Review, 22*(3), 310–314. doi:10.2307/2088472

Tacitus. (n.d., April 21). *Annals*, Retrieved from http://www.britannia.com/history/docs/tacitus.html

Turner, B. S. (2007). The futures of globalization. In G. Ritzer (Ed.), *The blackwell companion to globalization* (pp. 675–692). Oxford: Blackwell.

Van Gennep, A. (2010). *The rites of passage*. London: Routledge.

Whyte, W. F. (1993). *Street corner society: The social structure of an Italian slum* (4th ed.). Chicago: University of Chicago Press.

Young, M. W. (1979). *The ethnography of Malinowski: The Trobriand Islands 1915–18*. London: Routledge & Kegan Paul.

Zinn, J. O. (2008). Heading into the unknown: Everyday strategies for managing risk and uncertainty. *Health, Risk & Society, 10*(5), 439–450. doi:10.1080/13698570802380891

Zinn, J. O. (2015). Towards a better understanding of risk taking: Key concepts, dimensions and perspectives. *Health, Risk & Society, 17*(2), 99–114. doi:10.1080/13698575.2015.1023267

Faith and uncertainty: migrants' journeys between Indonesia, Malaysia and Singapore

Loïs Bastide

In Indonesia, transnational labour migrations have become a major source of foreign currency over the past 20 years. On migration routes and abroad, migrants are often subjected to abusive, sometimes violent or even deadly experiences. Yet, the 'migration industry' can count on increasing numbers of candidates. Drawing on 20-month multi-sited ethnographic fieldwork conducted between 2006 and 2009 in Java (Indonesia), Kuala Lumpur (Malaysia) and Singapore, I explore how, under these circumstances, migrant workers relate to this risky adventure. As it appears, local conceptions of 'fate' help to overcome fear: as future is perceived in terms of destiny, and since destiny lies ultimately in the hands of God, dealing with potential risks is a matter of religious *faith*: only by surrendering sincerely to Allah is the migrant able to secure his or her future in this dangerous milieu. In this cognitive framework, incidents are conceived of as *cobaan Tuhan* – godly trials – full of meanings, which are meant to test one's faith in God. And bad experiences, rather than being seen as *contingent*, are perceived as godly signs, which need to be interpreted in order to comply with God's will. I aim to show how this worldview formulates risk and/or uncertainty in terms of *nasib* and/or *takdir* (fate; destiny). This relation to risk, in turn, challenges Western-centred risk theories in adding nuance to the relationship between agency and risk, by tracing a singular conceptual tension between risk and *fate*.

Introduction

In this article I explore how labour migrants who undertake transnational journeys deal with the uncertainty and danger of their voyage. Drawing on data from an ethnographic study of Indonesian labour migrants, I examine the ways in which they deal with the numerous uncertainties they face while in migration. Besides practices developed in order to control risks materially, through the use of social capital or informal insurance practices, I show that migrant workers also engage religious faith as a means of managing these challenges. My focus, in this paper, is on this latter type of risk thinking. I examine how religious practices relate to the use of concepts such as risk, and what this religious ethos tells us about risk theories. In conclusion, I come back to the relationship between material and religious means of dealing with risks, by proposing that risk-mitigation practices, in this context, can be conceptualised in terms of 'mixed rationalities'.

Risk and migration

Risk and rationality

In Indonesia, transnational labour migrations have grown steadily over the past 20 years. In 2010, there were six and a half million Indonesian citizens officially working across a dozen countries, mostly in Pacific Asia and in the Middle East. If we add to the picture the flow of irregular workers, which by nature is impossible to account for precisely but is sizeable by every estimate,[1] Indonesia counts among the five biggest labour exporters worldwide. These labour journeys are highly hazardous, as migrant workers are subjected to abusive, sometimes violent or even deadly experiences. In these senses, *dealing with risks* is thus a critical component of migration experiences. Yet, this aspect of migration tends to remain somewhat neglected and under-conceptualised within migration theories, or is considered only in peripheral ways.

Unsurprisingly due to the prominence of the concept of risk in economic theory, economists have tackled this intersection most explicitly by considering migration as a means of dealing with *risks to livelihood*, at the individual or at the household level (Massey et al., 1993; Amuedo-Dorantes & Pozo 2006; Agarwal & Horowitz 2002; Yang & Choi 2007). Within this tradition, risks are thought to be dealt with by individuals in terms of a calculative balance between potential threats and benefits in the context of decision-making processes related to migration projects; these decisions are analysed based on rather simplistic models of rationality (Williams & Baláž, 2012).

In the fields of sociology and political science, however, the relationship between risk and migration has mainly been dealt with in more nebulous ways. Few studies have foregrounded risk as an explicit conceptual problem. Among those, some studies deal with risk-pooling strategies in migrant social networks (Mazzucato, 2009), while other research tackles the fact that taking risk provides positive identity attributes, as referred to for instance in the 'lifestyle migration' literature (O'Reilly & Benson, 2009). Another strand of inquiry has focused on the government of migration, with many authors stressing the increasing framing of migration as a *security* issue (see for instance: Bigo 2002; Faist, 2006; Huysmans 2000; Neal 2009; and for Indonesia: Arifianto 2009). Even if risk as a concept is not discussed in its own right, these analytical frameworks deal with the construction of migration as a *societal risk*.

In the context of Southeast Asia, researchers have drawn on the concept of governmentality to stress the unequal distribution of social vulnerabilities across the political body according to nationality, ethnicity, gender, religion and occupation (see for instance: Ford, 2006; Garcés-Mascareñas, 2008; Kaur, 2004; Piper, 2008; Silvey, 2006; Yeoh, 2006). For example, Aihwa Ong has identified the consolidation of 'graduated citizenship' (2006) and 'variegated sovereignty' (2008) regimes in Asian tiger economies, which organise the vulnerability of migrants across the region. A differentiated and unequal 'risk landscape' can therefore be inferred from these studies.

Besides this literature, some ethnographic studies have reversed the focus by looking at the various ways in which migrants *cope with* the threats faced while migrating across the region: by designing specific spatial practices (Silvey, 2004; Yeoh et Huang 1998); by developing border crossing strategies (Lindquist, 2009); or by using illegality as a means of avoiding exploitative labour relations (Killias, 2010). All of these types of research deal indirectly with risks, yet they do not consider risk as a specific topic and they do not discuss it as a core conceptual issue.

Given these gaps, in this article I focus explicitly on risk as a conceptual problem by looking at risk-mitigation practices in the context of regional migrations in Southeast Asia. I will examine how Indonesian migrant workers negotiate, individually and collectively, their relationship to the many uncertainties throughout their journeys. I will show that in this social setting, individuals relate to impending threats in terms of *fate*. Rather than contingent, potential harm is perceived as pertaining to destiny. And this belief in destiny raises an important issue: given this conception, can we speak of *risks* considering that '(a)s long as the future is interpreted as either predetermined or independent of human activities, the term "risk" makes no sense at all' (Renn, 1992, p. 56)?

Using this social-constructionist view of risk as a starting point (Zinn, 2008a; Lupton, 1999) is interesting because it allows a more fine-grained definition of the term: rather than taking the existence of risks for granted, it supposes that risk is a specific way to frame reality. Thus, in order to talk about risks, several criteria have to be met: First, the future must at least be seen as partly undetermined, otherwise risk turns into fate. Second, it must be perceived in terms of threats and possibilities. Last, these threats and possibilities must necessarily be correlated with human activities, otherwise no risk can be attributed to any course of action. It is only when these three conditions are met that we can think of a social subject that undertakes risk calculation to frame practical engagements.

This conceptual framework is useful since it breaks down the concept into several sub-components and opens up the possibility of distinguishing between different strains of risk thinking according to the specific articulations between these three criteria. It means that we need to look at actual practices in order to unravel the kind of relations they express regarding the future, what modes of framing threats they reveal, and whether or not these threats are dealt with using specific strategies. In this respect, by locating risk in a social setting where the future is perceived in religious terms, the case of Indonesian migrant workers raises several interesting issues.

As Le Breton (1995) phrases it, 'The notion of risk involves distancing from an existential metaphysics and refraining from seeing behind events the mark of a divinity rather than the play of circumstances' (my translation, Le Breton, 1995, p. e1). This highlights a central assumption of risk theories: that 'risk thinking' is a type of rationality which draws a clear line between incompatible ways of representing the future. Accepting this assumption means that the traditional world of superstitious or religious practices and conceptualisations is classified as irrational. In this *episteme*, future is not apprehended as a space opened to human agency and action but as fate; as a consequence, the future is met with passivity. On the other hand, we would have modernity (often equated with 'Western civilisation') with its forms of calculative rationality, where risk participates in the colonisation of the future as Giddens asserted: 'The notion of risk becomes central in a society which is taking leave of the past, of traditional ways of doing things, and which is opening itself up to a problematic future' (Giddens, 1991, p. 111). In this historical process, the future is seen as a partial outcome of human praxis and it is considered amenable to human action through various individual and collective forms of prudential practices, giving rise to the 'risk society' (Beck, 1992).

As with every clear-cut conception, this neat analytical distinction between risk and destiny, rationality and tradition, should raise a healthy dose of suspicion for any empirically minded social scientist. Having said that, my hypothesis is that in the context of my fieldwork and social scientific approaches to risk, we face 'mixed forms' of rationality that do not match this binary divide. If risk is related to a certain conception of the future as amenable to human action, there we find *another form* of risk thinking that needs to be qualified.

Migration routes: manufactured uncertainties and lived experiences of vulnerability

Since the late 1960s in Singapore and since the 1980s in Malaysia, transnational labour has been mobilised on an increasing scale and through increasingly formalised channels (Kaur, 2007). Foreign workers have been used by successive governments in both countries to establish a position and secure a position within globalising economic geographies. In the two 'developmental states' (Castells, 1992; Low, 2001; Olds & Yeung, 2004), it was a way of securing economic growth and promoting the fast development of a middle class that was to form core political clienteles for so-called 'semi-authoritarian' regimes (Ong, 1999). This government-driven social mobility resulted in labour shortages in the lower segments of labour markets, as nationals moved toward more qualified jobs. At the same time, shortages of reproductive labour in the domestic sphere also became pervasive, as policies were developed to increase the enrolment of women citizens in labour markets. Last, and more broadly perhaps, discrepancies between economic and demographic growth contributed widely to the need for labour imports (Drabble, 2000). In both countries, the influx of migrant labour was used by the state to ease these tensions: 'guest workers' have thus been used to supply those segments of labour markets abandoned by nationals and have been mobilised as a market-oriented solution to a new demand for labour in the domestic sphere. As a whole, this transnational labour force has enabled Malaysia to retain its niche position within the 'archipelago economy' (Veltz, 1996) by providing cheap labour for offshore production.

As this development model was established over the past 30 years, Malaysia and Singapore's dependence upon transnational labour has grown steadily; in 2011, estimates put the total number of foreign workers in Malaysia at anywhere between 2 and 4 million, or between 18 and 30% of the total employed labour force of 12 million. In Singapore, 544,700 transnational workers were recruited to feed low-skilled jobs, out of a total workforce of 3,443,700 (17%) in 2013. Thus, migrant labour has gradually become a centrepiece of governmental policies, as it has allowed the lowering of tensions between the social costs of neoliberal economic policies aimed at integrating global economic circuits, partly by attracting transnational corporations, and the fostering of national populations. In this context, migrant workers have absorbed most of the damaging effects of Singapore and Malaysia's developmental strategies, as they constitute the segment of the population most immediately exposed to neoliberal discipline – highly exploitative labour relations – and, as non-citizens, to the harshest effects of the biopolitical ordering of the national body[2] – as the 'foreign other' of consolidating national identities. In this position, guest workers are subject to cross-cutting sets of contingent practices, somewhat self-consciously designed by governments, which intersect and result in their confinement within segregated physical, social and political spaces.

Conversely, in Indonesia, labour exports have become a major source of foreign currency and a sizeable economic sector with total remittances of up to 7.4 billion US dollars in 2013, a figure that does not take into account the recruitment and placement business, which is a highly lucrative economic sector involving recruiters, financial institutions and transport (Bastide, 2015a). Overall, labour exports have thus become a critical economic sector, backed currently by a comprehensive institutional environment. They are now promoted as an important part of the country's export policies and are being integrated in bilateral trade agreement negotiations through commercial attachés in Indonesian embassies. In other words, migrant workers have been politically 'manufactured' as commodity exports. Moreover, related policies have tended to subordinate the organisation of their safety and protection to this economic role.

As these specific needs and uses in the three countries were increasingly institutionally entrenched, Indonesian workers became an important piece of an aggregating transnational political economy. Because Malaysia and Singapore relied increasingly on these migration flows, it was important to secure both their influxes and the specific qualities of this labour: its price and servility. Obviously, none of these 'qualities' are natural to these circulating populations, even though they are often represented as such in destination countries: that is, they need to be 'manufactured'. Additionally, migration routes – understood as specific social spaces – have played a critical role in this respect. Without entering into too much detail, two important points need to be made about the organisation of these labour flows: first, these transnational circuits articulate different places that display characteristics of 'disciplinary institutions' (Foucault, 1975) – spatial confinement; spatial and temporal partitioning (*quadrillage*); and policing. Second, they are the outcome of complex linkages between official, unofficial and criminal networks.

When migrant workers enter migration routes, they are thus 'circulated' between different 'transit houses' – *penampungan* – where they wait for a calling visa or to be transferred to another 'labour broker'; training centres, where they receive a minimal education for their future job; their workplaces in destination countries; and, sometimes, immigration detention centres. In all these locations, they usually undergo harsh disciplinary practices – bodily constraints such as mandatory haircuts for women, the inculcation of specific postures and attitudes or, in the worst cases, sexual abuses; the imposition of rigid spatial and temporal grids; compulsory confinement; and other such practices. This results in workers being subjected to derogatory regimes of citizenship on migration routes and to disciplinary processes that would not be conceivable under the umbrella of full citizenship entitlements in all three countries. In addition, these disciplinary processes often end up in heightened forms of violence in the workplace in destination countries.

Regarding the second point, the intricacy among official, unofficial and criminalised migration routes make them highly *unpredictable* for migrant workers. Migration routes are made of regular, irregular or criminal segments, which can be articulated in long chains (Bastide, 2015a). Migrant workers can thus be traded between different business partners, and there is little room for these workers to guarantee their final status in destination countries: opting for the legal process, in Indonesia, is by no means a guarantee that one will end up in a regular situation in Malaysia and Singapore. Conversely, choosing an unofficial route can end up in a regular situation as a documented worker. More fundamental to the discussion perhaps, whatever their final status as workers, migrants are often subject to more – in Malaysia – or less – in Singapore – drastic forms of institutional and interpersonal violence.

When we combine these characteristics, two things become apparent: first, that migrant workers are often exposed to diverse forms of moral and physical, and institutional and interpersonal violence, which make migration a fateful journey. Widespread moral and sometimes physical violence unfolds in transit houses as in the workplace.

Cases of migrant workers – especially transnational domestic workers, an exclusively feminine job – subjected to deadly violence by their employer are commonplace stories in the Indonesian press. Workers are also subject to institutional and social violence. In Malaysia, national and municipal police forces, immigration officers and state-sponsored militiamen repress migrants' presences and visibility in public spaces (Bastide, 2014; Garcés-Mascareñas, 2008; Wong & Anwar, 2003). In both countries, degrading stereotypes ascribed to migrant workers among national citizens deploy other forms of symbolic violence, causing moral wounds. For women, migration routes sometimes end up in 'karaoke bars' or in brothels along Indonesian frontiers (Ford, 2006; Lindquist, 2009), in Malaysia or in the City-State. Furthermore, risks related to migration do not only lie in destination countries. Potential mishaps also plague a possible return to home societies: long stays abroad threaten the integrity of marital relations; they often irremediably impact affective relations among family members; and more broadly, transnational journeys threaten one's position within the community, as social and cultural expectations toward returning migrants reshape their social position in their home places (Bastide, 2013). In short, transnational routes form a very dangerous or 'risky' milieu.

The second point is that migrants are usually fully aware of these traps and dangers. However, again – and this is critical to the discussion – many of them have little means of controlling these threats; that is, their fate in this complex social milieu is ridden with a deep, barely reducible *uncertainty*. Therefore it makes sense to examine these migrations in terms of an analysis of risk and related approaches for coping with uncertainty (Zinn, 2008a).

Methodology

In this article I draw on data from an ethnographic study of migration in Southeast Asia. The backbone of my investigative methods was the practice of a multi-sited ethnography (Falzon, 2009b). Between 2006 and 2009, I conducted fieldwork in a village in Central Java (Indonesia), where I spent more than a year; in Singapore, where I spent two months, following migrants in their daily life, and working in several NGO settings; I did the same in Kuala Lumpur (Malaysia), where I stayed for six months. Following migrants across different locations and in different social settings and activities enabled me to capture migration experiences *as they unfolded*, by observing practices rather than by relying only on retrospective verbal accounts of life in home communities (if doing ethnography in destination countries) or in migration (if locating fieldwork exclusively in the region of origin). It also allowed me to analyse transnational practices, experiences and social ties in their different 'local settings'.

On a more epistemological note, engaging in a multi-sited strategy is justified by two important assumptions: (1) that the pertinent social context of these migrations is *transnational* by nature. Indeed, if we take seriously the epistemological axiom that space is both a product of, and a context for, social practices (Lefebvre, 1991; Massey, 2005), then the proper contexts for analysing transnational migration are necessarily *transnational spaces* (Bauböck & Faist, 2010; Levitt & Schiller, 2004; Portes, Guarnizo & Landolt, 1999; Vertovec, 2009); and (2) more broadly speaking it is also true that if we are to 'follow [actual] practices' (Marcus, 1995), then we end up acknowledging that *all* social practices have varied spatial ramifications, that exceed the local contexts of their effectuation. Doing multi-sited ethnography is a way of acknowledging this property of the social which concerns not only the specialised domain of migration: even if it does not forbid the development of 'uni-sited' research strategies (Candea, 2009), this important consideration prevents looking at societies as sets of socially and spatially self-contained 'social worlds'. Multi-sited ethnography, in this perspective is thus a way of avoiding 'methodological holism' (Falzon, 2009a) by returning to a radical pragmatist perspective on social practices and experiences (Dodier & Baszanger, 1997) that illuminates their many spatial ramifications.

By sticking again to a pragmatist epistemology, I was able to examine the ways in which practices (including discursive practices) and cognition were embedded in specific social settings: in the ethnomethodological vocabulary, they are radically *indexical* (Garfinkel, 1967). Thus, the way social subjects relate to their social experiences is highly context-sensitive. So what is captured through the observation of actual practices (including discursive practices, again) is highly dependent on the location of the ethnographies: what we collect, while getting people to speak of their migration experiences back home, for instance, is not only a proxy of actual experiences abroad. It is largely, perhaps, an objectivation of how people relate to their past according to the necessities of their *current* social experience, *back home*, which is very different (Bastide, 2015a).

My first line of ethnographic inquiry was then combined with in-depth biographic interviews with migrant workers: understanding migration experiences requires the recovery of their many, interlaced, temporalities, since migration means dealing with varied *time-spaces* (Tarrius, 2010). These interviews were used in order to develop this diachronic perspective through the reconstruction of migration 'careers' (Becker, 1963; Glaser & Strauss, 1971; Goffman, 1971). I conducted 28 interviews in Indonesia, 18 in Malaysia and 14 in Singapore. In doing so, I faced two main challenges:

In these social contexts, individuals are not used to considering themselves as individuals abstracted from the collective – a prerequisite of many biographic sociological techniques, where a subject is asked to reflect on his or her *individual* experiences and expectations, as a discrete subjectivity (Bastide, 2015a). Due to vernacular forms of individuation, personal stories are always told as narratives of collective trajectories – involving collective goals, expectations and experiences. Individuals are thus displayed as *participants* in a common project rather than *subjects* of an individual life. In order to overcome this bias, biographic interviews were thus shaped as 'practices narratives' (Bertaux, 2005), which do not require the institution of an individual subject of an individual story but ask for more neutral practical descriptions.

Furthermore, interviews raise the issue of the 'attitudinal fallacy' (Jerolmack & Khan, 2014), understood as the inadequacy between information released in the context of an interview and real practices. Accepting this criticism means acknowledging that discursive contents produced in this context are, at least in part, outcomes of the condition of the interview as a specific social setting: this auto-referring bias casts doubts on the ability to draw factual elements from this method. In order to start to control this limitation, I conducted interviews within the social networks which I investigated through ethnographic practices. This triangulation of methods (Apostolidis, 2003) had several consequences.

First, it allowed the framing of interviews according to previously collected biographic information gathered in the course of less formal ethnographic relations. I was thus able to rely on 'thick' social relations, developed with interviewees in the course of multiple interactions. Common experiences in different social settings had brought us to know each other through different social identities (Goffman, 2005) and roles (Hughes, 1984), in more or less formal settings, from NGOs to karaoke bars. By developing, diversifying, aligning and deepening common knowledge and expectations, these ongoing relations broadened the scope of interview situations from often overly narrow social contexts, as they were linked to many common experiences located in other spaces and times.

Combining ethnographic practices and interviews provided a cross-perspective on individual trajectories (Bastide, 2011): through more or less formal speech acts, such as chats in the course of shared situations or interviews; through the variety of observed practices; and through the collection of a variety of reciprocal knowledge circulating within social networks. In the village, for instance, individual narratives were thus put in perspective according to different accounts from friends and relatives.

On a more theoretical level it is also useful to stress that that it is important not to presume on the adequacy between discourses and practices, but it is also difficult to assert the absence of relationship between the two. The real difficulty is that discourses do not refer transparently to the practices they narrate. As sense-making devices, they always have a temporal bias (Weick, Sutcliffe, & Obstfeld, 2005) as they read past events according to the current necessity of action. They always operate under an imperative of accountability (Garfinkel, 1967). Thus both dimensions make these discourses highly sensitive to current circumstances (hence the attitudinal fallacy criticism). A critical methodological problem is thus the issue of *referentiality*: discourses do not faithfully stage the practices they describe. Rather they *make sense* of practices, according to current circumstances, in order to *prepare for action* (Weick et al., 2005).

Given these observations I will start the consideration of my data by orienting my analysis to one fundamental consideration: the risk-taking practices of migrant workers who leave in spite of the highly uncertain outcomes of their journey and their risk-taking behaviour *in migration*, as they repeatedly take very uncertain bets on their well-being. I will then look at the ways individuals *make sense* of these attitudes by analysing associated discourses on risks. I will finally return to practices in order to show that, depending on the uncertainties of specific situations, discourses on risk are related to different types of actions and, more specifically, to different forms of risk-mitigation practices.

But prior to this discussion, a last point must be made about the discursive material which I will draw upon: its apparent gender bias. Indeed, the paper draws mostly on quotes taken from interviews with women. That is because women have always proved more willing to speak in an interview setting. I do not have time to dig into this issue, but this fact is easily explained (see Bastide, 2014, 2015a). For one thing, they thus provided more articulate insights in terms of 'risk thinking'. Moreover, there is a gender bias in terms of an individual's exposure to risks. Due to their involvement in certain sectors of labour markets (such as domestic work), due also to gender inequalities and stereotypes in Indonesia as in destination countries, women do indeed face a *riskier* journey than their male counterparts. In this sense, they are more expert at dealing with risks. However, I am confident that religious attitudes towards risks were similar across genders.

Findings

Migration and religious response to danger and uncertainty

Considering migrants' experiences of commodification and violence and the hazardous nature of migration routes, it is clear that migrants are undertaking a major gamble when they decide to migrate. Of course, the strength of their impetus to venture abroad is hard to deny and is based on various economic and social reasons, some comparable only to the extent that they combine to set actors into motion. However entrance onto migration routes, as a social process, is far from exhausted by these incentives: the relationship to an uncertain future and the potential threats which are thereby revealed, are also salient. More specifically, fundamental questions are put forward by the sheer number of actors willing to opt for this dangerous journey *in spite of* obvious threats – for movement and *risk* rather than a conservative but safe immobility.

Many migrants start on the migration routes, whether under-age, using fake identities and/or through notoriously dangerous channels such as irregular placement companies or informal placement networks, with little or no guarantee for their safety. Many also keep on repeating hazardous decisions even though past individual or collective experiences have proved these to be dangerous. Decision-making processes thus appear to proceed without proper risk assessments based on established knowledge from their own experience, from family members or community memories. However, at the same time migration also gives place to a broad set of prudential practices developed to reduce possible hardships, showing that those involved are well aware of the risks they face and that they do try to reduce them *to an extent*. Contrary to what could be suggested by the apparent absence of a relationship between available information on potential threats and decision-making processes, these practices show that we cannot reject bluntly the idea that we are faced with a *particular form* of risk thinking. These practices take different forms.

In Banyu Putih – the Javanese village where the Indonesian fieldwork was located[3] – as in other places in Indonesia where no previous culture of migration existed, domesticating the uncertainties related to migration has involved cultural innovations, developed in order to make sense of these new social experiences. Thus traditional propitiatory practices have been repurposed to counter pending threats and to summon good fate upon migrants. Among other instances, Javanese ritual meals – *slametan* – are now routinely organised before departures to try and ensure migrants' safety. By reaffirming and strengthening the traditional collective order in front of these new, disruptive transnational experiences (Bastide, 2015b), this ritual aims at safeguarding the harmony of the orderly village – *desa diatur* (Bertrand, 2003, p. 297) – in a time of tremendous changes. The dominant perception in the community is that participating in these meals is a way of acknowledging their allegiance to the universe of traditions and engaging benevolent forces to take care of the migrants on their journey. These innovations not only involved Javanese magical practices – known as *kejawen* – but also reinvestments of religious beliefs[4]: under certain conditions, the *act of leaving* has come to be considered as an efficient way of securing transnational trajectories, as the courage it involves, being conscious of related risks, is perceived as a display of religious faith. As they shape discourses and subjectivities, these cultural innovations provide insight into practices that on initial consideration would appear to be risk-blind. Nita, a young woman in her early twenties who worked as a domestic worker in Singapore, shed light on this point in the following way:

> I was brave enough to leave [to migrate] because I surrendered my fate to the Almighty. It strengthened my will. Finding a job, working, life and death, I entrusted everything to the Almighty.

This logic of justifications frames most of migrants' narratives. The trope of a delegation of responsibility to God – *Tuhan; Yang Kuasa; Allah* – to which migrants surrendered their fate – *pasrah* – played a critical role in shaping and fulfilling the will to leave. Through this course of action (the act of leaving), individuals did indeed comply with a central religious tenet, as their boldness was read as an act of *faith*: entrusting one's life and death in God's hands, by taking this dangerous journey, was a powerful way of proving the depth of their religious commitment.

In turn, this relation between the act of leaving, as a risk-taking behaviour, and religious faith, can only be established through a certain cultural relationship to the future, understood as *fate* or *destiny*. As Ari, a 26-year-old domestic worker in Singapore said[5]:

> Many people leave Indonesia … from my village to work abroad. Many are working abroad. In fact … I looked for information first: Which life do we live there? You see? People say that it depends on fate. On Allah. If your fate is good, you will end up in a good situation, you will be successful. But otherwise … you have to accept. What else can we do? Success … success depends on fate. Going there means being dependent on fate. So everything depends on fate … on Allah. Some get a good employer, some end up with a bad one. Some … before … images of employers having raped their employee … rapes, tortures … we often saw that on TV, in papers, you see? I left full of fear. But when I recalled life in the village, what else could I have done? [6]

As this quotation makes clear, this understanding is linked to the framing of the future as the domain of God. Future does not unfold out of pure chance or through the concatenation of mundane determinants, but as a *fatum*, which is the expression of Allah's will. As a result, the uncertainties of migration experiences are not conceived of as related to a contingent nature of events, but to the opacity of God's intentionality. It is only when this conceptual context – the relationship to existence as fate and to fate as an attribute of God – has been established that the act of leaving, as a display of religious faith, can be analysed.

The sociological dynamics operating here can be clarified using Goffman's concept of 'character' (Goffman, 2005). Indeed, given the fact that the decision to leave is *problematic*, since it represents a jump into 'something not yet determined but about to be', and since it bears potentially very serious consequences, because life is at stake, it can be understood as a 'fateful situation', in Goffman's term (2005, p. 153). Goffman shows that fateful situations are where one's *character* can be assessed according to one's composure in facing risk, except that here character attributions are not the product of an interaction between an actor and a mundane public assessing his or her action: they lie in the relation between a religious subject and God. Therefore, what is assessed is not character as a social, but rather as a *religious* quality: the valued religious subject is the one able to surrender to the Almighty in a context where he or she takes conscious risks, thus proving the depth of her faith. And this act of embracing one's destiny retains its own normativity since its quality is evaluated according to the *sincerity – keikhlasan –* of one's surrendering, which should be void of afterthoughts. Through this *sincere surrendering*, expressed in the act of leaving, a religious subject recognises the future as God's domain. Nika, a 27-year-old domestic worker, in Singapore, illuminates this point:

> I went to Jakarta, to Bandung. She [her friend] told me: 'little sister, do you want to enroll in the PT [recruitment agency]? Let's go to Saudi.' 'Where is Saudi?' I told her. 'Ah! We are going to make a lot of money in Saudi.' 'But I am ... afraid! I told her. 'What am I going to become?' 'Just entrust yourself – *pasrah* – in God's hands. Then you will be looked after'.

Sincerity of religious commitment was thus perceived as a display of religious character and a means, through this display, of summoning God's benevolence upon oneself by demonstrating one's compliance with religious precepts, thereby securing one's future. Quite paradoxically, taking risks was thus perceived as a means of avoiding risks; proving one's fate in the Almighty was understood as a way of seeking God's shelter.

The mobilisation of religious resources allowed social actors to restore – or safeguard – a sense of their own agency. Indeed, religiosity involved a broad range of possible attitudes and practices that allowed migrants to perceive themselves as *active* rather than passive beings in confronting potential threats. It was nevertheless also the case that the practical usefulness of religious resources could be legitimately challenged from the perspective of more familiar risk-mitigation practices. Putting oneself in the hands of God, it can be argued, actually pushes migrants to take unconsidered risks such that, rather than preventing potential threats, it has the opposite effect of *increasing* risks and risk-taking behaviours.

Risk, agency, responsibility

Whatever the actual outcome of these practices in terms of an actual exposure to risk, it is worth stressing that they indicate a belief in the possibility of affecting the future, as one's action, because it is submitted to godly judgement and has effects on the later unfolding of a destiny. Nowhere is this more obvious than in the vocabulary of migrants who consider leaving home a way of *challenging their destiny – mengadu nasib*: fate is not a given and should not be met passively. It is something one has to actively engage in, in order to fulfil its full virtualities. As Appadurai noted that risk is a cultural way of framing the future – the future being a *cultural fact* – (Appadurai, 2013), and after the implication of Zinn's observation that 'the concept of risk is tied to the possibility that the future can be altered – or at least perceived as such – by human activities' (Zinn, 2008a, p. 4), then the migrants in this study are engaged in a particular form of risk thinking. As I have shown, the main difference with this way of framing risk compared with the usual framing in sociological studies is that the *source* of uncertainty does not lie in the contingent nature of a mundane world deprived of intentionality, but originates in the opacity of God's will. If we recognise this common concern with risk, it is important to consider as well the very distinctive theoretical and practical forms this concern takes, in the context of this vernacular conceptualisation of uncertainty.

On a practical level, this understanding of existence as destiny and of destiny as a prerogative of God affects the relationship between a subject and his or her future, not so much because it drives migrants into thinking that they will be spared the misfortunes of migration, by putting themselves in God's hands, but rather because they accept that they should confront the traps dispersed on migration routes as a religious necessity – the unavoidable product of a *fatum* that an individual has to embrace as Allah's mark upon their life. Moreover, with destiny being acknowledged as the domain of God, its forms were conceived of as an expression of his intentionality. For a religious subject, the proper behaviour thus brings an individual to embrace their fate as a testimony of their faith but also as a *meaningful trial*: putting oneself sincerely in God's hands is a means of recognising, ensuring and clarifying that all the difficulties one will have to face are not a form of divine punishment, but rather a fruitful engagement with God's will, a lesson, a path for improving one's quality as a religious subject. As for Lidia, a 26-year-old runaway maid in Singapore, for many migrants these conceptions sustain attitudes of acceptance, underpinned by religious beliefs:

> Now let's hope if God allows me to ... I mean ... My goal now, let's hope that the Almighty allows me to ... that I can move on without obstacles ... move on ... move on. Maybe all that is just a trial for me. I must be patient, patient, patient [laughs]. And because we keep this patience in our hearts ... In order to obtain what we seek we have to pray, to keep on praying to God. And always be patient.

This attitude of acceptance also raises the issue of the relationship between the individual and her capacity to act, as Lidia seemed to defer action by entrusting her future with God. This issue was made even more acute by Nami, a 28-year-old domestic worker in Singapore:

> When someone asks me 'what is your goal? What are you looking for?' I mean ... why don't I rebel against my life? My answer is always the same: 'I only follow the stream'. Like water. If we follow the stream we will be happier. If we oppose it becomes more difficult. The stream, if we follow, at some point ... between the deep forests it will stop, and maybe we will find the right place. Thus I do not rebel. I ... I accept everything.

As with Lidia, Nami recognised and clarified the necessity to comply with fate (captured in the metaphor of the *stream*). What was at stake, as a result, was the attribution of agency in a context where Nami seemed to relinquish her own intentionality. This attribution is important because the possibility for a subject to conceive the possibility to act upon the future is a *sine qua non* condition of a risk culture: if we assume that it is characterised by a prudential relation to the future, it supposes the existence of an individual *responsible for* her own action and able to organise it so as to reduce risks. One's moral qualities as a responsible individual can then be assessed or debated according to the practices one develops to modulate one's exposure to future threats. However, such responsibility only makes sense if, and only if, we consider the individual as an autonomous source of action. This piece of speech – as in the case of Lidia's – can create the impression of a passive being, whose action, or lack of, is determined by heteronomous forces. It thus suggests an important question: if one's actions are determined by a transcendental volition that one has to comply with, are we still in the presence of a *subject* capable of autonomous action? Additionally, if God is considered the genuine source of action, are we still in the domain of risk thinking at all? Interestingly, however, Nami adds:

> [With] People it is different. If we do not oppose, they trample us [laughs]. People, we have to oppose. What I cannot oppose is my fate. I never oppose. I follow the motion. Against people yes! I often oppose! [laughs]

Taken together, these quotes sketch a 'moral economy' (Fassin, 2009) of action where acting seems to be expected on the part of the individual, yet under particular conditions and modalities that need to be specified. Importantly, it shows that it is important not to conclude that, in this particular context, the responsibility of the individual in relation to his or her action is diminished: rather, it is displaced. In this high-risk context, this responsibility is not assessed so much through the evaluation of an individual's practices developed to control materially the conditions of their exposure to risks. Certainly, 'following the stream', as Nami put it, can be considered in itself a certain type of individual agency, which requires a good dose of composure and equanimity and, more broadly, of personal engagement when facing difficult situations. However, it should not be confused with any form of classical risk calculation. This attitude does not rely on the undertaking of a 'reasonable' trade-off between risks and potential benefits, which would allow distinguishing recklessness from boldness. Rather it entails accepting a given situation as a necessity, whatever the risk it imposes on the individual. Recklessness is not seen as a failure to evaluate risks but rather as a failure to sincerely entrust one's existence to God. Yet it is important to stress that this way of coping with the neutralisation of individual and collective capacity of action regarding the threats of migration does not dissolve individual and collective agency. Rather, it frames it in a different way.

Destiny and sense-making

As I have pointed out, the deliberation that precedes the decision to leave does not start the future migrant questioning him- or herself in a mundane meditation over his or her own future; rather it puts him or her in the position of facing a divine will, expressed in the lines of a destiny. Complying with this will implies a range of related attitudes, expressing compliance by accepting the circumstances that Allah imposes upon oneself, which one should not fight but accept – *nrima*: the vagaries of existence are conceived of as godly trials – *cobaan Tuhan* – that should not be avoided nor met with revolt, rebellion or even reluctance. Rather, they require patience – *kesabaran* – both *nrima* and *kesabaran* being highly valued personal qualities in Java. The responsibility of the religious subject, in this context, is to *understand* the meaning of these trials, conceived of as clues that need to be decrypted to engage in the *right course of action* that is thus suggested in the mundane world by a transcendental will. Mariam, a young woman then in her mid-twenties, had worked as a domestic worker in Kuala Lumpur. At the time I met her, she was sheltered by an NGO after she had fled her employer. In itself, this excerpt is interesting: it shows that she relates to the hardship she went through as godly signs, which call both for acceptance and a search for meaning.

Researcher: You were deported from the country. But then how about the money you had saved in Malaysia?

Mariam: Yes, it was lost.

Researcher: Where did you keep it?

Mariam At home. In my home. I put it in clothes. Ok! It is my friend who took it, a thousand or two thousands [ringgits]. If I count ... Yes, it would be about 12 millions in Indonesian money. But forget it. Maybe because ... because I had gained this money this way ... yes ...

> maybe … maybe I did not have the right to use this money. Maybe I had had enough like this.

Researcher: You took it as a twist of fate?

Mariam: Yes. It is fate.

She added:

> Finally … my life was made of ups and downs. We were responsible together for our love [speaking of an old boyfriend]. But a lot of my difficulties related to… When life was good, he would make problems. He was like that. Finally when he hit me I accepted. Maybe it was my fate. And maybe it was a clue for me … about the meaning of my life.

In a context where the *right* principles of *a good* action, understood in religious terms, are conceived of as external to the individual, Mariam allows us to see the other side of the coin: this apparent passivity combines with an *active* interpretation of situations: complying with God's will requires an hermeneutic engagement on the part of the individual, which seeks to decipher meaning in the flux of his or her experience by elucidating the signs through which it is expressed. We are thus obviously dealing with an ethic of action, stripped from personal intentionality. To this extent, it echoes strongly the 'moral economy of volition' outlined by Bertrand (2003, p. 285), who shows that, in Java, subjectivation does not involve the affirmation of a subject *through* the manifestation of a personal will; it rather relies on a dissolution of personal intentionality and the opening of *ego* to the forces of an 'invisible world' – *dunia kang samar* – through ascetic practices.

However, at this point, it should be clear that this depersonalisation and this de-centring of intentionality does not imply a cultural representation of the individual as a passive being. It is true that the individuals perceive themselves as being dominated by destiny. However, they experience their power of action elsewhere: through their capacity of attention and their aptitude to decipher and decrypt the signs disseminated on their path, but also in their ability to take advantage of the elusive openings of a destiny according to these clues. What emerges then is this somehow uncanny situation where submission to destiny needs to be perceived as an *active practice*, which requires a continuous engagement. This oscillation or tension between individual action and its transcendental determinants outlines vernacular concepts of the individual. As Puspa, a 19-year-old young woman whom I met in a shelter for runaway maids in Singapore, commented:

> [Speaking about migrant women as a whole] From my point of view … Yes … as I said: it depends on fate. If their fate is good, they can succeed. If it is not good … just like me. It depends on fate … Yes … It depends on them alone actually! It depends on themselves, it depends on fate. Fate without struggling it cannot work.

Puspa provided another analytical step: she showed that there was room for both individual agency and an overarching transcendental will. More importantly, she showed that fate is not a given. To have a good life, one has to be up to the trials God imposes upon oneself, thus displaying one's quality as a religious subject. For one to be able to prove this religious quality, there has to be an autonomous sphere of action where one can express and show one's *own value*. Andi, a 31-year-old irregular mason in Kula Lumpur could thus say:

Andi:	Today it is true that many among the young do not have jobs. Like my friend … some do not know how to do but … They want to create a business, but what business he doesn't know. He is just sort of waiting … I don't know if he waits for destiny to fall down on him from the sky … For many it's like that.
Researcher:	They wait for wealth to fall from the sky …
Andi:	They wait but nothing comes.

Andi perceived destiny as relying both on a transcendental will and on the possibility of an autonomous sphere of practices, where a subject has to *take responsibility* for his or her own actions. Moreover when someone *is given* the opportunity to engage in material risk-mitigation practices, his or her responsibility is to do so since this chance is not seen as contingent, but as a meaningful opening. In this conceptual framework, future is thus constructed as being *partly amenable* to individual action. It is perceived as only weakly predetermined because it is thought that the personal qualities (or lack thereof) expressed through one's actions when facing godly trials will affect the latter unfolding of one's destiny – God rewarding a rightful action. Destiny, as a particular framing of the future, is thus best conceived of as a semi-open space for individual agency.

In this context, proving a genuine religious faith is understood as a way of mitigating risks. As I have shown, it involves three different levels of action: it takes the form of a display of religious character, a sincere surrendering. Furthermore, individual agency is displaced on the double level of a sense-making practice; it is expressed in the search for hidden signs in the unfolding of one's mundane experience as well as in the ability to trigger courses of action according to this interpretive work, in the context of a world represented as *consubstantial* to God's will. Destiny, as a cultural way of relating to the future, is thus obviously very different from mundane understandings of the future as a contingent space, stripped from transcendental volition. It is true also that the nature and definitions of risks vary greatly in these two different *epistemes*, physical risks being subordinated to religious risk in the Javanese context. However, both cases illustrate a sustaining of a sense of uncertainty, the giving way to conceptions of the future as partly amenable to individual action, and the making of room for practices aimed at reducing one's exposure to *risks*.

Conclusion: risk and mixed rationalities

Fate should not, therefore, be seen as opposed to risk; rather, it is understood as a specific space, the limits of which cannot be expanded, but within which individual agency can unfold and impact on the future of the individual. In a context where migrants are widely deprived of material possibilities of control over their becoming in transnational spaces, faith is then perceived as the only means of securing existences. Sincerity of surrendering – *ikhlas, pasrah*, patience in facing obstacles – *sabar*, being alert to signs, hermeneutic practices and the ability to catch opportunities to engage in proper courses of action are the type of practices that aim to comply with God's will, by struggling to living up to one's destiny. More critically, these are ways of pre-empting the future by means of one's own actions. However there is a very real risk of falling back into an old-fashioned culturalism. I would like to conclude by offering a few more empirical clues on how to steer clear of this pitfall.

As I have already noted, few social, economic or political devices are available for migrants to take and retain control over their transnational trajectories. In this context, the practices and conceptualisations that I have outlined must be understood as the *only available means* for many migrants to restore a sense of agency in facing serious threats to their health and well-being. In a context where current economic conditions and emerging moral economies render migration increasingly necessary, facing risk is less of a choice than a necessity. And this creative use of cultural resources allows making this relation between threat and necessity morally bearable when there is little choice but to engage in migration routes, regardless of the risk.

However, it is worth noting that more conventional risk-regulation practices (for risk theory) can also be observed among those few workers endowed with more resources, or benefiting from more favourable circumstances. Indeed, experienced migrants in Kuala Lumpur and Singapore are sometimes able to negotiate their whole trip without ever entering the migration industry; this can include the search for their own employer and can involve the negotiation of their work contract. Some migrants develop an *actuarial* relation to migration: in this case, making sure that one is always ready for a further round on migration routes is a way of dealing with unforeseen risks, by offsetting potential costs with the possibility of a new period of work abroad. In Kuala Lumpur, undocumented migrants secure their presence in the city by leveraging resources in their social networks in order to stay hidden or, for instance, to be informed about police raids. Recognising these mundane forms of risk-mitigation practices is important; however, it should not bring us to reduce the importance of more immaterial risk-management patterns, by considering it a second-best option, because if more skilled migrants develop other means of controlling their trajectories, they nevertheless also refer to and follow these religious prescriptions. What I want to suggest is that these two forms of engagement with risk are not exclusive – related to a magical or religious *ethos*, on one hand, and to risk-mitigation practices closer to more mundane forms of practical rationalities, on the other hand. They rather coexist, as migrants tend to develop *all available means* to secure their existences. As soon as circumstances, resources or skills allow it, individuals thus develop *both* material and religious means of controlling risks, as taking advantage of the opportunity of developing material risk-mitigation practices is also seen as a way of complying with God's will.

Given this, reflecting on the articulation between discourses on risks and actual contexts of action is critical: it shows that practices are at least as much determined by situational constraints as by ingrained interpretative schemes. And when migrants have the opportunity to engage in material risk-mitigation practices, it is interesting to see that material prudential attitudes develop. It is true nevertheless that this cultural relation to potential threats has powerful practical effects if we consider that it makes people much more prone to risk-taking behaviours. In highly uncertain situations where material risk-mitigation practices are not available, faith helps people engaging in high-risk courses of action, while retaining a sense of agency. In this context, prudential practices are thus inscribed in a wider conception of reality where natural and supra-natural forces are seen as composing a unified world, under the overarching gaze of God, and where religious, magical and material means of controlling risk are conceived as efficient.

It seems highly plausible that similar forms of 'mixed rationalities' (rather than the all too usual irrational vs. rational analytical pattern) related to risks exist in 'Western' countries (Zinn, 2008b). In the case of France, Favret-Saada (1977), for instance, has shown the persistence of magical practices. Numerous surveys also show the pervasiveness of beliefs in supra-natural forces and a widespread engagement in propitiatory practices, including avoidance of certain situations (like 13 people around the table) or uses of lucky charms. More broadly, faith in the future, even in a secularised perspective, is not an uncommon motive in the context of decision-making. On a more theoretical level, Zinn (2008a) notes that '(...) in [the] perspective of everyday life, risk is often calculated by intuitive or pre-rational techniques'.[7] Considering this, there is a need to depart from formal and normative definitions of risk thinking, as a type of rationality in its 'pure' or ideal form, to dig into the complexities of actual individual and collective practices aimed at gaining a degree of control over the future.

In doing that, one may well discover that 'mixed rationalities' are not only bound to 'traditional societies' (as opposed to 'modernity'). Rather they are a widespread means of dealing with risks in everyday life *as soon as life becomes uncertain* to the point that it neutralises the efficacy of material risk-mitigation practices. Starting amidst practices, one could well discover also that risk thinking, as it is often referred to in the literature as a purely calculative and utilitarian relation to the future, could be understood at best, with a sympathetic state of mind, as a Weberian ideal type rather than a good descriptor of actual practices. In a more critical spirit, it can be perceived also as a normative concept that is too theoretically abstract to account for actual practices beyond the calculative rationalities of institutions – insurance or the 'precautionary principle' (Ewald, 1996), for example. By restoring the thickness of these 'mixed rationalities', there is a chance we can devise a more anthropological description of risk as a *cultural fact*.

Disclosure statement

No potential conflict of interest was reported by the author.

Funding

This paper draws on research which has been funded by an 'Aire Culturelle' grant from the French Ministry of Research and Education, and by a research grant from the National Centre for Arts and Crafts, Paris.

Notes

1. In 2010, in Malaysia, the estimated number of irregular workers matched the official flows.
2. In both countries, the constitution and consolidation of a national 'imagined community' (Anderson, 1991) is a source of concern for political elites, in recently formed countries. These processes of 'nation building' have relied and resulted, albeit under different guises, in the ethnicisation of national societies in Malaysia and Singapore. In these contexts, foreign labour causes deep social anxieties in the two countries. This is perhaps especially true of Indonesian workers, who are often of the same ethnic stocks as Malaysian and Singaporean Malays (for an extensive account, see: Bastide, 2014, 2015a).
3. Banyu Putih is a small municipality located in the Special Territory of Yogyakarta, Java, in Indonesia. Home to about 2000 people, 80–90% of all households have or have had one of their members working abroad.
4. As with many anthropologists, I agree that we should distinguish between the magical and the religious: in short, I understand magical practices are a form of practical logic (as opposed to theoretical logic) linked to a religious world view (Keck, 2002).
5. All names are pseudonyms.

6. The last sentence of this quotation, where she expresses an imperative to migrate, should be interpreted with caution. In a context where migration is difficult to justify on the grounds of individual motives, especially for women, narratives of the decision to leave are constructed conventionally in the terms of a necessity, usually referring to the livelihood needs of the family (Bastide, 2015a). However, when the discussion is *oriented towards* the reasons behind a departure, these conventional justifications often fade away behind more intimate motives. Ari indeed is among those women whose decision to migrate, even if she had to justify it by arguing the will to improve her family's economy, was motivated by a refusal to conform to social expectations and available social roles, back in her village. Leaving was a way to open up new possibilities.

7. However, I hope to have shown that the risk-mitigation practices I have described are, in fact, perfectly rational in the cognitive reality they inhabit.

References

Agarwal, R., & Horowitz, A. W. (2002). Are international remittances altruism or insurance? Evidence from Guyana using multiple-migrant households. *World Development*, *30*(11), 2033–2044.

Amuedo-Dorantes, C., & Pozo, S. (2006). Remittances as insurance: Evidence from Mexican immigrants. *Journal of Population Economics*, *19*(2), 227–254.

Anderson, B. O. G. (1991). *Imagined communities: Reflections on the origin and spread of nationalism*. London: Verso.

Apostolidis, T. (2003). Représentations sociales et triangulation: enjeux théorico-méthodologiques. In J.-C. Abric (Ed.), *Méthodes d'étude des représentations sociales* (pp. 13–35). Saint-Agne: Erès.

Appadurai, A. (2013). *The future as cultural fact: Essays on the global condition*. Vols 1–1. London, Royaume-Uni, Etats-Unis: London. New York, NY: Verso.

Arifianto, A. R. (2009). The securitization of transnational labor migration: The case of Malaysia and Indonesia. *Asian Politics & Policy*, *1*(4), 613–630.

Bastide, L. (2011). *Habiter le transnational: Politiques de l'espace, travail globalisé et subjectivités entre Java, Kuala Lumpur et Singapour* (Unpublished doctoral thesis). ENS de Lyon, Lyon.

Bastide, L. (2013). Migrer, être affecté. Émotions et expériences spatiales entre Java, Kuala Lumpur et Singapour. *Revue Européenne Des Migrations Internationales*, *29*(4), 7–20. doi:10.4000/remi.6606

Bastide, L. (2014). Globalizing Kuala Lumpur: Indonesian migrant workers, urban borderscapes and the production of metropolitan spaces. In N. Aveline-Dubach, J. Su-Ching, & M. Hsing-Huang Hsiao (Eds.), *Globalization and new intra-urban dynamics in Asian cities*. Taipeh: NTU Press.

Bastide, L. (2015a). *Habiter le transnational: Espace, travail et migration entre Java, Kuala Lumpur et Singapour*. Lyon: ENS Editions.

Bastide, L. (2015b). Troubles dans le local: Migrations transnationales et transformations culturelles à Java. *Critique Internationale*, *65*, 1.

Bauböck, R., & Faist, T. (Eds). (2010). *Diaspora and transnationalism: Concepts, theories and methods*. Amsterdam: Amsterdam University Press.

Beck, U. (1992). *Risk society: Towards a new modernity*. London: Sage.

Becker, H. S. (1963). *Outsiders : Studies in the sociology of deviance*. New York, NY: The Free Press of Glencoe.

Bertaux, D. (2005). *Le récit de vie: L'enquête et ses méthodes*. Paris: A Colin.

Bertrand, R. (2003). Un sujet en souffrance? Rcit de soi, violence et magie Java. *Social Anthropology*, *11*(3), 285–302. doi:10.1017/S0964028203000211

Bigo, D. (2002). Security and immigration: Toward a critique of the governmentality of unease. *Alternatives: Global, Local, Political*, *27*(1), S63.

Candea, M. (2009). Arbitrary location: In defence of the bounded field-site. In M.-A. Falzon (Ed.), *Multi-sited ethnography: Theory, praxis and locality in contemporary research* (pp. 25–46). Farnham: Ashgate Publishing.

Castells, M. (1992). Four Asian tigers with a dragon head: A comparative analysis of the state, economy and society. In J. Henderson & R. P. Applebaum (Eds.), *State and development in the Pacific Rim* (pp. 33–70). London: Sage.

Dodier, N., & Baszanger, I. (1997). Totalisation et altérité dans l'enquete ethnographique. *Revue Française De Sociologie*, 37–66. doi:10.2307/3322372

Drabble, J. H. (2000). *An economic history of Malaysia, c. 1800–1990: The transition to modern economic growth*. New York, NY: St. Martin's Press in association with the Australian National University.

Ewald, F. (1996). Philosphie de la précaution. *L'année Sociologique, 46*(2), 383–412.

Faist, T. (2006). The migration-security nexus. International migration and security before and after 9/11. In Y. Bodemann & Y. Gökçe (Eds.), *Migration, citizenship, ethnos* (pp. 103–120). Basingstoke: Palgrave Macmillan.

Falzon, M.-A. (2009a). Multi-sited ethnography: Theory, praxis and locality in contemporary research. In M.-A. Falzon (Ed.), *Multi-sited ethnography: Theory, praxis and locality in contemporary research* (pp. 1–23). Farnham: Ashgate Publishing.

Falzon, M.-A. (Éd.). (2009b). *Multi-sited ethnography: Theory, praxis and locality in contemporary research*. Farnham: Ashgate Publishing.

Fassin, D. (2009). Les économies morales revisitées. *Annales Histoire, Sciences Sociales, (6)*, 1266–1237.

Favret-Saada, J. (1977). *Les mots, la mort, les sorts*. Paris: Gallimard.

Ford, M. (2006). After Nunukan: The regulation of Indonesian migration to Malaysia. In A. Kaur & I. Metcalfe (Eds.), *Mobility, labour migration and border controls in Asia* (pp. 228–247). Basingstoke: Palgrave Macmillan.

Foucault, M. (1975). *Surveiller et punir: Naissance de la prison*. Paris: Gallimard.

Garcés-Mascareñas, B. (2008). Old and new labour migration to Malaysia: From colonial times to present. In M. Schrover, J. Van Der Leun, L. Lucassen, & C. Quispel (Eds.), *Illegal migration and gender in a global and historical perspective* (pp. 105–126). Amsterdam: Amsterdam University Press.

Garfinkel, H. (1967). *Studies in ethnomethodology*. Englewood Cliffs, NJ: Prentice-Hall.

Giddens, A. (1991). *Modernity and self-identity: Self and society in the late modern age*. Stanford, CA: Stanford University Press.

Glaser, B. G., & Strauss, A. (1971). *Status passage*. London: Routledge & K. Paul.

Goffman, E. (1971). *Asylums. Essays on the social situation of mental patients and other inmates*. Harmondsworth: Penguin books.

Goffman, E. (2005). *Interaction ritual: Essays in face to face behavior*. New Brunswick, NJ: Aldine Transaction.

Hughes, E. C. (1984). *The sociological eye : Selected papers*. New Brunswick, NJ: Transaction Books.

Huysmans, J. (2000). The European Union and the securitization of migration. *JCMS: Journal of Common Market Studies, 38*(5), 751–777.

Jerolmack, C., & Khan, S. (2014). Talk is cheap: Ethnography and the attitudinal fallacy. *Sociological Methods & Research, 43*(2), 178–209. doi:10.1177/0049124114523396

Kaur, A. (2004). Crossing frontiers: Race, migration and border control in Southeast Asia. *Diversity in the Asia Pacific Region and Europe, 6*(2), 202–23.

Kaur, A. (2007). International labour migration in Southeast Asia: Governance of migration and women domestic workers. *Intersections: Gender, History and Culture in the Asian Context, 15*. Retrieved July 8, 2015, from http://intersections.anu.edu.au/issue15/kaur.htm

Keck, F. (2002). Les théories de la magie dans les traditions anthropologiques anglaise et française. *Methodos. Savoirs Et Textes*, (2). Retrieved July 8, 2015, from https://methodos.revues.org/90

Killias, O. (2010). Illegal migration as resistance: Legality, morality and coercion in Indonesian domestic worker migration to Malaysia. *Asian Journal of Social Science, 38*(6), 897–914. doi:10.1163/156853110X530796

Le Breton, D. (1995). *La sociologie du risque*. Paris: PUF.

Lefebvre, H. (1991). *The production of space*. Malden, MA: Blackwell.

Levitt, P., & Schiller, N. G. (2004). Conceptualizing simultaneity: A transnational social field perspective on society. *International Migration Review, 38*(3), 1002–1039.

Lindquist, J. A. (2009). *The anxieties of mobility: Migration and tourism in the Indonesian borderlands*. Honolulu: University of Hawaii Press.

Low, L. (2001). The Singapore developmental state in the new economy and polity. *The Pacific Review, 14*(3), 411–441. doi:10.1080/09512740110064848

Lupton, D. (1999). *Risk and sociocultural theory: New directions and perspectives*. Cambridge: Cambridge University Press.

Marcus, G. E. (1995). Ethnography in/of the world system: The emergence of multi-sited ethno-graphy. *Annual Review of Anthropology, 24*(1), 95–117. doi:10.1146/annurev.an.24.100195.000523

Massey, D. B. (2005). *For space*. London: Sage.

Massey, D. S., Arango, J., Hugo, G., Kouaouci, A., Pellegrino, A., & Taylor, J. E. (1993). Theories of international migration: A review and appraisal. *Population and Development Review, 19*(3), 431. doi:10.2307/2938462

Mazzucato, V. (2009). Informal insurance arrangements in Ghanaian migrants' transnational net-works: The role of reverse remittances and geographic proximity. *World Development, 37*(6), 1105–1115. doi:10.1016/j.worlddev.2008.11.001

Neal, A. W. (2009). Securitization and risk at the EU border: The origins of FRONTEX*. *JCMS: Journal of Common Market Studies, 47*(2), 333–356.

O'Reilly, K., & Benson, M. (2009). Lifestyle migration: Escaping to the good life? In K. O'Reilly & M. Benson (Eds.), *Lifestyle migration: Expectations, aspirations and experiences* (pp. 1–13). Farnham: Ashgate.

Olds, K., & Yeung, H. (2004). Pathways to global city formation: A view from the developmental city-state of Singapore. *Review of International Political Economy, 11*(3), 489–521. doi:10.1080/0969229042000252873

Ong, A. (1999). Clash of civilizations or Asian liberalisme? An anthropology of the state and citizenship. In H. L. Moore (Éd.), *Anthropological theory today* (pp. 24–47). Malden: Polity Press.

Ong, A. (2006). *Neoliberalism as exception: Mutations in citizenship and sovereignty*. Durham, NC: Duke University Press.

Ong, A. (2008). Scales of exception: Experiments with knowledge and sheer life in tropical Southeast Asia. *Singapore Journal of Tropical Geography, 29*(2), 117–129. doi:10.1111/j.1467-9493.2008.00323.x

Piper, N. (Ed.). (2008). *New perspectives on gender and migration : Livelihood, rights and entitle-ments*. London: Routledge.

Portes, A., Guarnizo, L. E., & Landolt, P. (1999). The study of transnationalism: Pitfalls and promise of an emergent research field. *Ethnic and Racial Studies, 22*(2), 217–237.

Renn, O. (1992). Concepts of risk: A classification. In S. Kimsky & D. Golding (Eds.), *Social theories of risk*. London: Praeger.

Silvey, R. (2004). Power, difference and mobility: Feminist advances in migration studies. *Progress in Human Geography, 28*(4), 490–506. doi:10.1191/0309132504ph490oa

Silvey, R. (2006). Geographies of gender and migration: Spatializing social difference. *International Migration Review, 40*(1), 64–81. doi:10.1111/imre.2006.40.issue-1

Tarrius A., (2010). Les nouveaux cosmopolitismes migratoires d'une mondialisation par le bas. In N. Bancel, F. Bernault, P. Blanchard, et al. (Eds.), *Ruptures postcoloniales: nouveaux visages de la société française* (pp. 414–428). Paris: La Découverte.

Veltz, P. (1996). *Mondialisation, Villes et Territoires: L'économie d'archipel*. Paris: PUF.

Vertovec, S. (2009). *Transnationalism*. London: Routledge.

Weick, K. E., Sutcliffe, K. M., & Obstfeld, D. (2005). Organizing and the process of sensemaking. *Organization Science, 16*(4), 409–421. doi:10.1287/orsc.1050.0133

Williams, A. M., & Baláž, V. (2012). Migration, risk, and uncertainty: Theoretical perspectives. *Population, Space and Place, 18*(2), 167–180. doi:10.1002/psp.663

Wong, D., & Anwar, T. A. T. (2003). Migran Gelap: Indonesian migrants in Malaysia's irregular labour economy. In G. Battistella & M. B. Asis (Eds.), *Unauthorised Migration in Southeast Asia* (pp. 169–227). Manilla: Scalabrini Mirgation Center.

Yang, D., & Choi, H. (2007). Are remittances insurance? Evidence from rainfall shocks in the Philippines. *The World Bank Economic Review, 21*(2), 219–248.

Yeoh, B. S. A. (2006). Bifurcated labour: The unequal incorporation of transmigrants in Singapore. *Tijdschrift Voor Economische En Sociale Geografie, 97*(1), 26–37. doi:10.1111/tesg.2006.97.issue-1

Yeoh, B. S. A., & Huang, S. (1998). Negotiating public space: Strategies and styles of migrant female domestic workers in Singapore. *Urban Studies, 35*(3), 583–602. doi:10.1080/0042098984925

Zinn, J. O. (Éd.). (2008a). *Social theories of risk and uncertainty: An introduction*. Malden, MA: Blackwell.

Zinn, J. O. (Éd.). (2008b). Heading into the unknown: Everyday strategies for managing risk and uncertainty. *Health, Risk & Society, 10*(5), 439–450. doi:10.1080/13698570802380891

Applying the risk society thesis within the context of flood risk and poverty in Jakarta, Indonesia

Roanne van Voorst

Scholars have called for further critical reflection on and hence advancement of popular theories of risk. Classic texts such as Beck's risk society thesis have been criticised for their Eurocentricity, making them difficult to use in non-Western contexts. This limitation is especially problematic given that so many risks and natural hazards occur in precisely the Southern, developing regions of the world which Beck's work largely neglects. In this article, I draw on data from a year of anthropological fieldwork (2010–2011) plus shorter follow up visits to the research area in 2014 and 2015. I use these data to examine the relationship between Jakartan slum dwellers' experiences and perceptions of severe, recurrent flood risk and the central arguments of Beck's thesis. I argue that while some elements of Beck's theoretical framework provide insights into a non-Western, highly risk-prone context, other aspects of his thesis are less helpful and need to be reworked using alternative theories of risk.

Introduction

In this article, I critically review the utility and suitability of Beck's risk society theory for examining the ways in which an extremely poor and flood risk-prone community of riverbank settlers in Jakarta, Indonesia, perceive and manage the danger of flood risk. Beck developed his theories as way of explaining how and why risk has become so important in late-modern (high-income) societies. Through the processes of globalisation, he also argued that this late-modern structuring of risk spread to low-income countries. In this article, I examine the extent to which Beck's theories explain how vulnerable individuals living in low-income countries respond to the threat of natural disasters.

The applicability of the risk society theory outside late-modern society

Beck, in his risk society thesis (1992, 1995), claims that, while modern societies have developed a fine-grained set of institutions and regulations that divide and manage wealth and growth, they have failed to develop institutions that deal with the risks that characterise late modernity. As a consequence, the traditional industrial class structure of society is breaking apart, with the development of 'risk society' in which social conflicts no longer centre on class or the division of wealth, but instead centre on the division and management of risk. The defining characteristic of this 'new modernity' is not 'the distribution of goods', but 'the distribution of bads': who is exposed to which risks, who is able to protect him/herself from risks and who carries responsibility for risks? Over the years, Beck and several proponents of his thesis have developed what became widely known as the reflexive modernisation school – which I will discuss in more detail later in this article.

In recent years, Beck's thesis has been subject to major criticism from a range of social scientists (see Mythen, 2007), who have argued that the thesis is Euro-centric and only loosely based on empirical evidence. Many scholars have questioned whether Beck's key arguments are valid for understanding risk experiences in non-Western or developing regions.

A starting point for an examination of the relevance of Beck's theory to risk in more traditional societies is a more detailed analysis of his theories and in this section I focus on four key elements of his theory:

- New (manufactured) versus old (natural) types of risk.
- The democratisation of risk and its separation from the class structure and hierarchy so that risks are 'democratic' rather than class-hierarchical.
- The globalisation of risk with 'cosmopolitan events' impacting on people living in the non-Western, most risky parts of the world.
- The politicisation of risk through contested risk claims.

The changing nature of risk: new versus old risks?

In his risk society thesis, Beck highlights the changing nature of risk production in late-modern society. While such societies produce the same risks that afflicted industrial society, such as industrial pollution and natural disasters, they also create new invisible, invisible risks – for instance, in the domains of health, food and pollution. As such risks are globalised, they cross social, cultural and generational boundaries. Traditional hazards tended to be local, personal and time bound, for example, a hunter being injured during a hunt. The new risks of late modernity, such as global warming, are not bounded by place, person or time (Beck, 1992, p. 22–23; Beck & Beck-Gernsheim, 2002, p. 41; Luhmann, 1993, p. 89–95). The impact of nuclear disasters such as Chernobyl stretches across frontiers affecting individuals who have no connection with the accident such as sheep farmers in the English Lake District. They are not time-limited – they affect the health and well-being of future as well as current generations.

Beck differentiated 'natural' hazards or dangers, which he associates with traditional society, from 'manufactured risks', which he argued characterise late-modern society. Commentators have criticised this classification of risks pointing out that man-made 'risks' occurred in early, traditional societies, for example, the hazards associated with living in small huts with smoky fires in close proximity to animals, while some 'new' risks are so complex that it is difficult to neatly conclude whether they are man-made, caused by a chain of events, or by phenomena we do not yet understand (see Anderson, 1997, p. 188; Furedi, 2002). This argument is, in fact, older than Beck's thesis. Already in 1976, Phil O'Keefe, Ken Westgate and Ben Wisner published a landmark article in *Nature*, called *Taking the naturalness out of natural disasters*. More recently, researchers have showed that 'natural' hazards are always, to some extent, 'manufactured' (Blaikie, Cannon, Davis, & Wisner, 2004, p. 40). Mythen has argued that Beck's rigorous categor-isation may result in an underemphasis on the impact of catastrophic 'natural' disasters that still occur across the world (Mythen, 2007, p. 799). Alaszewski (2004) has also cautioned that focusing on the 'new' risks highlighted by the risk society debate may mean that scholars of risk forget about 'old' risks, which still have a major impact on late-modern society (2004, p. 3). Beck's attempt to link different types of risk to different periods of time is not always helpful for our understanding of human risk experience. Instead, risk researchers should take into account both 'types' of danger/risk and acknowledge that can and do occur in the West as well as in the non-West; in the so-called 'developed' regions of the world as well as in the developing regions.

Risk society and the (ir)relevance of class

Beck argued that many of the most pressing current risks are global in character and their impact is not shaped by the social and political class system that has formerly characterised industrialised societies. 'New' risks such as climate changes created by global warming are capable of cutting through traditional class-based distribution of benefits in society, as they will affect wealthy citizens as well as poor citizens. Beck, therefore, (in)famously contends that 'poverty is hierarchical, while smog is democratic' (Beck, 1995, p. 60) and that the dynamics of risk society bypassed social status and class because 'global threats ultimately affect everybody, even those responsible for them' (Beck, 2009, p. 22). Consequently, he argued that the manufactured 'bads' act as a trigger for political action in the global risk community. Highly concerned citizens will unite and try to diminish risk, for example, by challenging the risk knowledge of authorities and experts. I will elaborate these 'politics of knowledge' later in this article but, at this point, it is helpful first to reflect on the implication of this following Beck's theory. Essentially Beck noted that it changes the nature of the basic concepts of sociology, including social class, but also of power, and even of the state and the nation itself. Beck argued that social scientists should no longer focus on social class but should move their attention to the 'global social constitutive conditions of risk' (Beck, 2009, p. 52).

However, other sociologists have argued that Beck overstressed the change and claim that social class remains an important aspect of contemporary society (e.g. see Atkinson, 2007; Goldthorpe, 2002; Mythen, 2005, 2014; Scott, 2002). They maintain that risks are distributed along lines of wealth and power; and risks are shaped by social class. Curran has asserted that class has become *more* important to an individual's life chances with the growing emergence of a risk society (2013, p. 46). While Beck noted that risk knowledge is constantly contested by different actors in society (suggesting that these actors have the agency to do so), the anthropologist Mary Douglas argued that dominant groups in society decide what is risky or dangerous, and who is to be blamed for when there is a failure to predict and manage risk. In any given society, risk is contested and the outcome of such contests is shaped by power, class and group status (e.g. insiders vs. outsiders).

Beck responded to such criticism by refining his analysis of the relation between risk and class. In 2010, he acknowledged that 'new' risks impact on individuals around the world in unequal ways, thereby exacerbating inequalities between the rich and the poor. However, he argued that such inequalities are only evident for individual risks, such as disease, not for systemic risks such as climate changes or air pollution. Wealthier people can buy protection against and treatment for individual risks, which poorer people cannot. He maintained that systemic risks disregarded class inequalities (Beck, 2010, p. 165). He thus maintained his view that 'class' had become 'too soft a category to capture the explosiveness of social inequality at the beginning of the twenty-first century' (Beck, 2013, p. 63).

Risk society and globalisation

Beck was convinced that 'new' risks such as environmental pollution could create global 'traumatic experiences' that somewhat equally 'threaten[ed] everyone's existence' – be they rich or poor; he also believed that this global experience would create a community of world citizens to ameliorate such global risks (Beck, 2009, p. 51).

However, as I have already noted some of his critics have argued that such a view of human risk and responses to them is Eurocentric. Although Beck described the current risk society as a global society, his analysis focused on the impacts of risk in Western capitalist cultures, mostly German and British (Nugent, 2000, p. 236). His assumption that people's risk perceptions and risk experiences are relatively homogeneous all over the world fails to pay attention to the differentiated nature of populations and the importance of social stratification in shaping vulnerability to and experience of risk (Mythen, 2014, p. 135).

As I have already observed disasters occur much more frequently in some regions than in others, then it seems unlikely that all humans around the world perceive 'risk' in similar ways. Rather, individuals are likely to have very different experiences of modernity – as well as of the risks that modernity produces. While an increased awareness of risk may be a novel outcome of the project of modernity in the eyes of a (Western) scholar, risk often has a less exceptional status for those at the periphery of modernisation processes. Those individuals who have to deal with immediate life-threatening hazards, such as floods, infectious disease and hunger, may be less interested or concerned about long-term abstract, universal risks such as climate change and environmental pollution (Nugent, 2000, p. 226).

Caplan, therefore, has suggested that analyses of risk need to take into account individuals' differential experiences of risk, and researchers need to focus in context rather than taking universal approaches (Caplan, 2000). There is evidence that the local experience of risk, combined with local social structures such as gender hierarchies and processes of inclusion and exclusion, leads to culturally specific interpretations of risk. Cultural attitudes towards risk are accordingly heterogeneous (Douglas, 1966; 1992; Douglas & Wildavsky, 1982; Weber & Hsee, 2000). Such evidence indicates that, rather than an approach that disregards local context, researchers need to examine the cultural and everyday contexts in which it is experienced and interpreted by different groups of people in different ways. Since Beck's thesis has seldom been applied to non-Western, developing regions, its relative validity within these risk contexts remains a moot point.

Furthermore, Beck's critics have argued that there is little evidence of widespread concern about global systemic risks such as global warming. For instance, Dickens (1992) has observed that while many citizens across late-modern societies are aware of the existence of systemic environmental hazards, they do not all necessarily believe that these risks affect them. Individuals can and do hold a range of ambiguous and contradictory views about these systemic risks. Dickens has claimed that Beck is simply projecting his own critique (and fears) of industrialised society onto the general population with little regard to what they actually think (Dickens, 1992, p. 12–17). Similarly, Giddens has suggested that while people are aware of global risks such as climate changes, the issue generally remains so abstract and vague to them that they do not feel any great concern nor do they feel the need to take action to decrease these risks (Giddens, 2009). Mythen has echoed this position, writing that 'inasmuch as the spectre of the global bads of the risk society….may occasionally filter across consciousness, many people are bound up with managing more humdrum risks: finding and keeping a job, paying the rent, having enough money to feed and clothe the kids...' (2014, p. 136).

Such criticisms suggest that the risk society thesis is not just Eurocentric but generally tends to overemphasise global citizen's concern with abstract risk. As a result, it largely fails to interrogate the importance – or otherwise – of large-scale risks within the wider construction of personal biographies (Mythen, 2014, p. 136).

Risk society, blame and responsibility: the politics of risk

In his thesis, Beck identified historical development that culminated in a society radically changed by experiences of untraceable risk. He argued that in premodern societies risks were essentially 'blows of fate' that threatened human beings from outside and were mostly attributed to external gods, demons or nature (Beck, 2009, p. 6). In contrast, he argued that in late-modernity risks are seen as the result of human decisions; therefore, humans are blamed for their negative consequences. At the same time, it is not clear who can be held formally responsible or accountable for universal systemic risks such as environmental pollution. He noted that the institutions of modern society acknowledged the existence of current global risks and sought to negotiate agreements and take actions to minimise these risks, but such agreements and actions tended to be ineffective. Beck argued that such failures stimulated new forms of politics. For example, increased debates conducted publicly by experts and lay people in mass media into the real or possible consequences of technical and economic decisions (Beck, 2009, p. 6). This new form of politics also included greater citizen participation in decisions on how to manage risks; given the complexity and contestation of knowledge about these new risks and given the desire of governments to transfer the responsibility for decision-making from the state to citizens.

Beck's thesis that new forms of risk have stimulated new forms of politics has been criticised both empirically and theoretically. Irwin and his colleagues (1999) showed in their empirical work on risk perception that Beck underestimated the level of contra-diction, incoherence and disagreement in the ways in which citizens make sense of risk. They argued that while citizens did derive some of their information about risks from expert sources most of it came from individual experiences, local memories, moral convictions and personal judgements (Irwin et al., 1999, p. 1312).

Beck was not attempting to provide a detailed account of the ways in which indivi-duals acquire and create conceptions of risk nor an empirical investigation of the complex reality of risk perceptions; he wanted to offer a critical view of the role that risks plays in late modernity. However, as Wilkinson has noted, any attempt to mask the complexity of the social experience of risk in rigid conceptual abstractions may lead further away, rather than closer to, a more intimate understanding of the day-to-day reality in which people experience risk (Wilkinson, 2001, p. 11).

Beck's assertion that new forms of risk are creating new forms of politics has been criticised on the grounds that there is nothing particularly new about risk in late-modern society. Beck argued that the 'new' technological-scientific hazards such as nuclear radiation underpinned the emergence to 'risks society'. However, Mary Douglas has argued there is nothing specially distinctive about 'modern' risk and has emphasised the similarities between human risk experiences in contemporary society and those in any other period in human history (Douglas, 1992, p. 11; Wilkinson, 2001, p. 3).

Douglas's emphasis on continuity is based on her cultural theory of risk that she articulated in her early work (1966, 1969) on purity and pollution. She argues these concepts are used to construct and maintain boundaries within and between social groups and between the self and other. The inappropriate crossing of boundaries creates pollution and dirt, substances in the wrong place, threatening social order and stimulating action to restore the boundary and avert the danger. Douglas described how the Hima people of Uganda believed that contact between women and cattle would result in cattle becoming sick and dying. Douglas argued that this set of beliefs functioned to reinforce the differentiation of gender roles, thus helping to maintain the social order (Douglas & Wildavsky, 1982, p. 40–48). She noted that beliefs about purity and pollution play a key role in creating the various social boundaries that underpinned the maintenance of social order (Tansey & O'riordan, 1999, p. 74).

Douglas argued that risk in modern secularised societies plays the same role as taboo and sin did in religious premodern societies (Douglas, 1990, p. 12). In contemporary Western society, concepts of purity and pollution are also used to define and maintain boundaries. These concepts are used to identify danger and to allocate blame, for example, in the racist 'science' of the Nazi, 'unhygienic' disease bearing Jews threatened the purity of the Germanic race. A 'risky' Other may threaten the individual member of a group or the symbolic body of the whole community. In order to maintain social order, communities therefore single out some objective hazards as risky, while disregarding others. The risks that are defined as dangerous, then, provide explanations for things that have gone wrong or unfortunate events that are deemed to threaten community (Douglas, 1992). While Beck argued that an emergent 'risk consciousness' was giving rise to a new form of politics and culture, Douglas argued that risk was a new name for a well-established phenomenon.

Evidence for this idea has been provided by scholars such as Mieulet and Claeys (2014), who, in their research on the risk of Dengue fever in Martinique and French Guyana, showed that mosquito control was to be used by societal groups as a means of overcoming social tensions between them by identifying a common external enemy that failed to recognise and take action against the shared threat presented by mosquitoes (Mieulet & Claeys, 2014, p. 595). This finding strengthens the point that risk perception and defined responsibility regarding risk prevention for a dengue fever epidemic are always related to broader sociopolitical issues and culture (p. 581).

Comment

There are four key elements of Beck's risk society thesis that have been subject to critical comments:

- new versus old risks,
- the (ir)relevance of class,
- universal versus context specific risk perceptions and
- the role that risk has come to play in society.

In this article, I will use data from an empirical case study of floods and flooding in Jakarta to explore the salience of Beck's relatively abstract theory of risk society to the everyday cultural processes and practices in one of the more risk-prone areas of the global South.

Methodology

The social context for testing the risk society theory

Different lists of 'the top 10' of most dangerous cities in the world exist, but Jakarta is mostly included in them; see, for example, Michael (2014). In Jakarta, residents live amidst the threats of severe, recurrent floods. It is therefore a good setting within which to examine the ways in which residents, especially those living in vulnerable areas, conceptualise and deal with risk.

In this article, I draw on the findings of 12 months of anthropological fieldwork (starting in 2010) that I undertook in one of Jakarta's poorest neighbourhoods, located alongside the banks of a branch of the Ciliwung River, the largest river in Jakarta. My research centred on the ways in which people dealt with floods and the factors underlying their risk behaviour. I selected this neighbourhood, which I call Bantaran Kali in this article, because it is one of the most flood-prone areas of Jakarta. Each rainy season there are floods that are at least 1 metre high that create economic losses and outbreaks of diseases. There are also exceptional floods that can be as high as 6 metres (Texier, 2008).

Approximately 3.5 million people live along the riverbanks of the Ciliwung in Greater Jakarta. Of these, 759 live in Bantaran Kali – 232 households (*Kepala Keluarga*). The residents have built their houses from wood, asbestos, plastic and stone. Whenever floods occur, these houses are inundated by contaminated river water, damaging people's valuables and exposing them to waterborne diseases. The floods worsen the economic situation of the poor, which in turn increases their physical vulnerability. They also cause fear and anxiety within the neighbourhood: even though many people in the community are to some extent used to living with floods and have found ways to cope with them, for example, through engaging in mutual help networks in the neighbourhood or by adapting their houses, floods are still considered by people as scary, problematic and worrisome.

Floods are particularly problematic for these riverbank settlers because the government offers no effective social safety net to support flood victims, while residents can themselves not afford to save large sums of money as a buffer that could be used in times of disaster. Most of them earn less than 50,000 Indonesian Rupiah per week (less than 5 dollars). This income is barely enough to pay rent, feed one's family and pay for children's school uniforms.

Ethnographic methods

My ethnographic fieldwork was a rich source of riverbank settlers' perceptions of, and experiences with, floods. I was able to use participant observation: living alongside the residents of Bantaran Kali to share their experiences and explore their understanding of the flood risk that characterised their daily lives. I rented a small room in the house of one of the residents, from which I slowly and gradually became familiar with my temporary neighbours' daily lives. During three floods that I experienced in the field, I was able to observe study participants' responses to them. These observations offered me data which I draw on in this article.

I supplemented the participant observation with more structured data collection. I obtained information about residents' perceptions of risks through a group interview exercise with residents, called 'risk mapping'. This risk mapping aimed to illicit residents own accounts of risks. Thus, rather than asking participants to rank or choose from a predetermined list of risks, I asked them to tell me about all the things that worried them in their neighbourhood: the things that threatened their safety, the problems they dealt with and the uncertainties that threatened their sense of well-being. This identification of problems can be thought of as a way of looking at the local perceptions of risk and it allows the researcher to understand which risks are given priority by the people who face them (Quinn, Huby, Kiwasila & Lovett, 2003). Barrett, Smith, and Box (2001) have argued that risk mapping offers a systematic but simple approach to classifying and ordering sources of risk faced by a group of people. In Bantaran Kali, 20 respondents (12 male and 8 female, 11 born in the area and 9 newcomers, aged between 19 and 71 years) participated in the risk-mapping exercise. In order not to steer their risk perceptions, I told the participants that my research focused on 'life in the kampong'. I asked participants to describe the different risks, problems or uncertainties in their lives and which they perceived as most threatening to their well-being. The participants identified a wide range of risk including floods, fires, evictions, becoming ill from typhus, losing an income or job, not having money to pay for one's medical treatment in case of illness, becoming ill from dengue fever, drowning and getting ill from the river water. I wrote all risks mentioned by residents during the group discussions on a large sheet of paper and invited participants to clarify them. For example, why did they consider floods in Bantaran Kali risky? Was it an economic or a health risk? To whom?

After participants had discussed each risk, I invited them to rank them in order from most pressing to least pressing. The participants' ranking indicated that there were two groups of danger that caused greatest concern for residents in Bantaran Kali: one group was based on the danger of floods but of nearly equal importance was a group of dangers relating to poverty such as sudden illness, a sharp decline in income or eviction from their house.

This grouping of dangers indicated that flood risk could and should not be treated in isolation. For the participants in my study, it was only one of the many risks they had to deal with in their lives. The discussion in the group interviews indicated that participants had to constantly balance a variety of risks and risk-oriented behaviours, for example, if their house was flooded would they seek safety on the roof of their house until it subsided hoping that their boss would understand their temporary absence from work, or would they try and swim through the currents – risking their lives but perhaps saving their job? It was clear from the discussion in the group interviews that flood risk and poverty-related risks could not be disaggregated. All the participants were exposed to flood risk because they could not afford housing in a safer, drier part of the city. Therefore, in order to study participants' risk experiences from a bottom-up perspective, I decided that it was necessary to take a broad approach to risk and include the pressing dilemmas and uncertainties related to poverty in my analysis.

This broad approach was most clearly reflected in the third and fourth methods that I employed: in-depth interviews and a survey. I carried out in-depth interviews with 130 respondents about their behaviours in relation to flood risk and poverty-related risks in their daily lives. I selected my informants on the basis of age (no people of under 18 participated in this study; the eldest was 67) and through snowball selection. More females ($N = 80$) than males ($N = 50$) participated; hence, there was a gender bias in the sample that may have affected the outcomes. Respondents were asked about what they perceived to be the cause of floods or other particular risks discussed in the interview, what they believed might be a solution to the risk problem, what were the effects of these risks on their well-being, who they thought should intervene to solve flood risk (or other risks that were threatening to the respondent) and how they personally coped with these risks.

I also carried out a quantitative survey on risk practices among the same group of 130 respondents. In the survey, 82 items were included that described common practices that people used to cope with flood risk, as well as 30 items that described common practices that people used to cope with poverty-related risks. Examples of flood risk responses were 'stocking food and water', 'building a ladder', 'evacuating', 'asking for financial assistance after a flood'; 'laminating valuable documents so that they cannot be damaged during a flood'; 'providing neighbours with food if they refuse to evacuate and have no food left in the house'; 'investing in social relations with actors who might offer financial support after a flood'; 'praying to Allah'. These items were either mentioned by study participants or referred to actions that I had seen people taking before, during or after floods. Study participants indicated which of the listed risk-handling practices they used, by answering yes or no. On the basis of these four sets of data (observations, risk mapping, interviews and surveys), I was able to interpret my participants' perceptions of risk, as well as to define patterns in their risk behaviour. I elaborate on these findings elsewhere (Van Voorst, 2014, 2015). In this article, I discuss those findings that shed light on the applicability of Beck's risk society thesis.

I interviewed around 20 government officials engaged in Jakarta's flood management, among which civil servants working for the city government and the municipality. This allowed me to crosscheck the information that I obtained from my study participants in Bantaran Kali about flood events, with formal information from authorities. In addition to this, I analysed policy reports and newspaper clippings from Indonesian newspapers that were relevant to the topic of floods.

Findings

Floods: a new or old risk?

The data from my fieldwork in Jakarta indicate that in this setting Beck's distinction between 'old' and 'new' risks, or between 'natural' dangers or 'manufactured' risks did not work. Participants in my study noted that floods in Jakarta are both an old and new problem; likewise, they are both natural and man-made.

In the view of my participants, floods are natural, in that Jakarta is highly flood prone due to its geographical location (Brinkman, 2009; Texier, 2008). For example, Tikus (male, 24) (all names in this article are pseudonyms) told me that 'this city is a dangerous place to live in, because so many rivers run through it. If you live close to them, like we do, you are threatened by floods all the time!' Participants also often referred to the fact that Indonesia's monsoons brought very intensive rainfall each rainy season (Marfai, Yulianto, Hizbaron, Ward, & Aerts, 2009). However, they also reflected on the 'manufactured' factors underlying the flood problems: urbanisation dynamics in Jakarta have led to more extensive use of the built environment, more garbage clogging the sewerage system and greater numbers of humans potentially affected. For example, Rian (female, 47) remarked that: 'this city is overloaded with people, and all those people throw their garbage in the river. I do that as well; what else can I do? There is no sewage system here! This city is a mess!'

As Rian indicates, rapid urbanisation is indeed one of the factors that has most severely aggravated the flood problem over time. In 1811, Jakarta had a population of about 47,000; today with a metropolitan population of more than 20 million and rising, Jakarta has become one of the world's largest cities (Cybriwsky & Ford, 2001; McCarthy, n.d.; Van Voorst & Hellman, Under Review). One consequence of such urbanisation has been that the city's governmental services have been put under increased pressure and cannot keep up with the demands of the fast growing population (Kadri, 2008; Sagala, Lassa, Yasaditama, & Hudalah, 2013). For example, more and more garbage clogs the sewerage system, and most of the city's former green space has now been built upon (Caljouw, Nas, & Pratiwo, 2005).

Ida (female, 45) said about this:

> It is impossible to stop floods here, because rich people have built too many factories and shopping malls over the past years in Jakarta. This pollutes the air so that we experience more rain, and therefore my house is flooded again and again.

While elite villas and shopping malls mushroom, state provision of housing for the poor has become inadequate relative to demand. As a result, many millions of poor inhabitants have moved into large informal settlements along Jakarta's waterways, rivers, reservoirs and sluices. These informal settlements contribute to the pollution and clogging of these flood-prone areas. In these senses, the social and the natural are closely intertwined within the generation of flood risk. I discuss the problem of informal settlement in more detail later in this article.

Floods are not a particularly 'new' problem either: admittedly, they are now increasing in volume and severity due to geographical, demographic, environmental and infrastructural reasons (Brinkman, 2009; Texier, 2008), but even during colonial times periodical inundations were already a rather common phenomenon in Jakarta (Caljouw et al., 2005).

Floods are (un)democratic

Beck's claimed that modern risks are 'democratic' in the sense that they cross social, cultural and generational boundaries. However, the participants in my study did not see the risks as democratic. Tikus said that:

> When large floods occur, the whole of Jakarta floods. But in this neighbourhood the floods are much more severe than elsewhere. For other residents of Jakarta, they are just a nuisance. For us, they can be a real danger – we often get ill from them and people sometimes drown!

Likewise, Ari (female, 36) told me that:

> in other parts of the city floods come only as high as your ankle or knee. Here, they can be metres high, so that people have to escape to rooftops in order to survive!

In the context of flooding in Jakarta, Beck's 'democratic' argument is only partly true. Some of the most severe floods affected over 70% of the city (Brinkman, 2009; Texier, 2008). These floods not only affected the poor river bank communities, but also the elite areas, located further from the rivers. This 'democratic' tendency of the flood problem is often highlighted in media accounts about floods in Jakarta. For example, a famous photo has been circulated on the Internet of the national president, his trousers up above his knees, in his flooded presidential house (Minuet of Life, 2013).

However, it needs to be emphasised that the coping resources of an elite flood victim such as the president, in comparison with those of poor river bank settlers, are very different. During large floods, the president might decide to reside on the 20th floor of one of Jakarta's many luxury hotels, or he might let his chauffeur drive him to his second house out in the countryside. In comparison, my informants have no option but to remain in their inundated houses for days or weeks. Elite flood victims also have the money to repair potentially damaged houses, to pay for medical treatment if they get ill from dirty flood water or to pay for health insurance. In contrast, my informants do not have such financial resources. What is more, they cannot make use of a formal social safety net, as this is not effectively provided by the state to Jakarta's poorest, and are therefore forced to cope with floods through autonomous coping strategies and informal self-organisation (I describe many of these strategies in more detail in Van Voorst 2014, 2015). Finally, it needs to be emphasised that in 18 years floods only seriously affected elite neighbour-hoods four times, while poor riverbank settlements such as my research area are flooded several times *each year*. At the time of writing this article, the most recent, severe floods had occurred in 1996, 2002, 2007, 2013 and 2014.

Beck's claim that risks nowadays cross societal lines of wealth and class therefore gives a very unrealistic idea of the flood problem in Jakarta. Rather, it can be concluded that experiences of flood risk largely follow the contours of class division in the city.

The relevance of abstract risk for actors in the non-Western world

Beck asserted that the risk society is global because wherever individuals live on the globe they are threatened by unknown, boundary-crossing risks such as climate changes or air pollution. As a result, citizens share concerns about such global, incomprehensible, abstract and unpredictable risks. Put in another way: they are to some extent unified by these risks. Other scholars have countered that global risks such as climate changes may not be relevant at all for people living in highly hazard-prone areas of the world (e.g. see Nugent, 2000).

Regarding the serious negative impacts of recurrent floods for Jakarta's poorest residents, one might expect that they are hardly concerned with abstract risks that are less pressing in their everyday lives. This was certainly my assumption when I began my fieldwork in the flood-prone, poverty-stricken area of Bantaran Kali. However, somewhat to my own surprise, I found while the participants in my study were most concerned with floods and poverty-related risks, at the same time they often expressed distress about global risks that – they believed – threaten their health and well-being, albeit in less visible or direct ways. For example, whenever I asked participants to tell me about the most pressing problems in their daily lives, they would typically mention acute problems such as floods, illness or poverty first, but then they would tell me about other concerns, such as climate change and air pollution. They associate such large-scale risks with the local flood problem in their neighbourhood. For example, Rian explained:

> Floods often occur here, but they also occur in other countries, did you know that? It is true, I saw a documentary about this some years ago on television. Everywhere there is air pollution because of how people treat the earth, and then all kinds of problems with nature arise. It worries me a lot: how can my children live a healthy life in such polluted world?

In a similar vein, Hassan (male, 66) recounted to me that:

> I am always concerned about floods. My family gets ill from them and our goods are damaged. It gives me a headache just to think about them! But if you ask me about other things that worry me...I am *very* concerned about climate changes. You know, the weather is acting funny nowadays, because people are not taking good care of the environment. (...) You can see the effects for yourself in this neighbourhood. We used to only have floods

during rainy season, but now, we have floods all the time. But other countries have similar problems. Like in the Arctic, the ice is melting? That is because of how humans treat the environment. You should be careful when you go back home to your country [the Netherlands], Roanne, because I have heard from the television that it might be flooded any time soon.

Participants in my study seemed to be aware of Beck's 'global risk society', in which people are unified in their concerns about cosmopolitan risks, and it is important not to dismiss this part of his thesis for people in non-Western societies too quickly.

Rian and Hassan indicated that riverbank settlers could and did access news items about global risks through television, and, in some cases, newspapers. The younger participants in my study had also learned in school about the issues of climate changes and air pollution – understandably a major issue in the smog-prone megacity of Jakarta. As a consequence, most river bank settlers were aware of these boundary-crossing and 'new' types of risks. In fact, it seems that their concerns about global, abstract risks such as climate changes were rather strong precisely because they associated them with a risk that is to them already very concrete: flooding.

However, as Jakarta's riverbank settlers were occupied with coping with flood risk in their daily lives they had scant energy left for *intense* worrying about more abstract problems – let alone for action to mitigate them (if effective action would be possible at all). In the words of Hassan:

> The world is a dangerous place that is what I think. The air that we breathe is not clean, in the future people might die because of that [pollution]. And if climate changes become worse, the seas will flood, the poles will melt. Scary, huh? Yeah, all these things concern me greatly, but I have no time to really think about them, to be honest with you [laughs]. I am always busy with cleaning up my house from floods, and with feeding my kids. I have no time for too many worries at once!

Other participants expressed similar views; they sometimes felt distressed about risks which some social scientists typically associate with late modernity but they were occupied with concerns about floods in their neighbourhood.

The politics of risk: blaming the victim

Beck contended that, in current risk society, what is perceived as a risk is constantly challenged by new or other types of information. Arguments about risk and risk policies are expressed in mass media, and overtly discussed in public. The result is that what is believed to be risky, and what should be done about it and by whom, is contingent and correspondingly is constantly challenged by different societal actors.

However, the findings from my fieldwork in Jakarta indicate that Beck's analysis of the 'politics of knowledge' seriously underplays the impact of the inequality of power in society. There was more evidence to support Douglas' approach and those commentators who stress the importance of social class and who argue that while risk knowledge may be contingent, only the most powerful actors are able to define the nature and source of risk. Such definitions attribute the blame to the marginalised powerless, in the case of Jakarta the riverbank dwellers who have 'chosen' to live in a dangerous area. Thus, in Jakarta, policymakers and city planners blamed those who lived in the flood plain for the harm that resulted from floods.

When I interviewed policymakers, they blamed the river bank settlers for floods, while downplaying or denying their own responsibility for solving the flood problems. Such narratives provided a justification for the minimal state support which flood victims received during or after floods. For example, one official blamed river bank dwellers in the following way:

> They built their houses on flood-plains! Of course they are flooded all the time! That is what flood plains are supposed to be for! We have floods because of those stupid *people*, not because of the river! So, no, of course I do not give them money after floods. It is their problem, they should solve it themselves.

Another official argued that 'We do not offer assistance during most floods in those neighbourhoods because they are not just flood-*victims*. They are actually more the *creators* of floods'.

As I have already noted, the participants in my study accepted part of the blame for the damage that resulted from the flood, though given their economic circumstances they felt they had no real choice but had to be in the wrong place at the wrong time. When asked about the causes of floods, most study participants mentioned their own residence on the river bank as one important contributing factor to the flood problem. In interviews, they recounted times in the past when the river banks were still green and uninhabited and told me that the river had become narrower, shallower and dirtier because they, together with so many others, built their houses on top of its banks. 'So basically', said Ida, 'we create floods ourselves, by living here'. However, participants also observed that they had no real choice, they could not afford to live in safer areas of the city. For example, Edi (male, 34) said:

> As long as people occupy the river banks, the city will be flooded. I live in this riverbank settlement, so I am co-creating floods. But there is no other place for me to live – other neighbourhoods are unaffordable for poor people like me.

Participants also blamed state officials who had both the resources and could use them to prevent the problems; for example, by rehousing them in a safe area. Tina (24) described the situation in the following way:

> Whenever there is a large flood in Jakarta, politicians always tell journalists that *we* are to blame. And I agree with them, actually. We built many houses on the river banks, therefore the river has less space than before. We also drop our garbage in the river, which clogs it. But sometimes I think: Why doesn't the government build houses for us in another neighbour-hood? All politicians spend money on is on more factories, more shopping malls, and more villas for the rich. While I'd love to live in a safe, dry area in Jakarta, but I cannot afford it. So if a journalist would ask me who to blame for floods, I'd tell him that floods are not just our fault but also the fault of politicians!

However, given the relative power relations between river dwellers and public officials only the voices of the powerful, the officials and politicians were reflected in policy documents and mass media reports, and these dominated both the public debate and policymaking on flood risk management. The voices of my participants were not acknowledged in public debate. Hence, Douglas' emphasis on the function that risk has in society (blaming, 'Othering', maintaining social order) seems most appropriate here. My findings show that in Jakarta the elite blame flood victims for floods, thereby shifting the responsibility for causing the flood problem from the state to the riverbank settlers.

This also implies shifting the responsibility in finding a solution onto the shoulders of the most marginalised.

While Beck suggested that such 'expert' views on risk can be effectively challenged by laypeople in society, there is little evidence for such challenging in Jakarta. The view is challenged by my informants but their opinion is not considered as 'true' or legitimate and correspondingly has no impact on risk policies.

Discussion

In this article, I have used empirical evidence from fieldwork in Jakarta to reflect on classic risk theory, especially risk society. As I have observed, Beck's risk society thesis has been criticised for its lack of validation in empirical research, as well as for its Eurocentricity. Moreover, various critics have questioned whether an overly narrow focus on risk may obscure other important issues such as power inequality and class. To this end, I have explored which aspects of the risk society thesis are pertinent and valid in the case of an Indonesian, flood-prone region, and which features would be better replaced or expanded through alternative theoretical perspectives.

One case study is not sufficient to make general statements about the usefulness of Beck's risk society thesis for risk studies in the non-West. My findings in Jakarta tell us little about the applicability of this theory in other hazard-prone regions of the South. Nevertheless, through my fieldwork I have been able to identify issues that are relevant for broader debates about risk theory.

Grand theories of risk are attractive because of their critical views of societal trends in risk consciousness rather than their ability to capture detailed conceptions of the social reality in which people acquire and create interpretations of risk. However, such a simplification of reality can obscure our understanding of human experience. The findings of the fieldwork in Jakarta show that some of the assumptions made by Beck about people's risk experiences and perceptions hold true in the case of Jakarta. However, there is still scope for further in-depth studies employing multiple methods to document the ways in which problems of risk feature in the everyday experiences of individuals and which draw on such evidence to critically engage with key risk theories.

Even though Beck's risk society thesis was developed in relation to (post-)industrialised, Western societies, the findings from my study indicate that some of its elements are helpful to explain how risk is identified, used and managed in other parts of the world. This means that, rather than developing a completely new risk theory for the non-West, and rather than dismissing the notion of risk altogether, it is helpful to elaborate and refine the central arguments of the reflexive modernisation framework in light of other issues that appear relevant to everyday lived experiences within risk contexts. In the case of Jakarta, it appeared that the topic of flood risk was interwoven with various issues of poverty and power inequality. A more holistic approach towards risk and uncertainty was therefore needed to reach a more adequate understanding of people's daily life experiences with risk. Rather than looking through a narrow 'flood risk lens', which restricts our understandings of people's risk experiences, it is important to adopt a wider approach to consider the range of risks identified by individuals and how they see them as relating to each other so that it is possible to see how specific risks such as those relating to floods are structured by and form part of wider risks such as those resulting from poverty and marginalisation. Rather than solely working with the notion of risk *or* replacing it for class, the findings of my study showed that it is most fruitful to use a theoretical framework that incorporates both issues – thus advancing a theory of risk, class and power. One example of such approach was recently provided by Mieulet and Claeys, who investigated the risk of Dengue fever in Martinique and French Guyana in relation to broader sociopolitical issues within different historical (heritage of colonialism and slavery), geographical (overseas territory) and cultural (ethnic diversity) contexts (2014, p. 582).

Conclusion

In a highly flood-prone and poor river bank settlement of Jakarta, residents were concerned with global risks such as climate change and air pollution. These concerns resemble the concerns of inhabitants of late-modern risk society, as described by Beck. However, it must be emphasised that rather than being concerned only with abstract risks, these residents were also and more seriously concerned with daily, pressing and very visible risks. Recalling the criticism of Dickens (1992) and Mythen (2014), it needs to be clear that a similar argument can be made for most people in the world (also those in Germany and the United Kingdom described by Beck), whose daily lives are perhaps not characterised by a risk as threatening as floods, but nevertheless filled with other types of problems, conflicts and threats that demand most of their attention.

Two elements of Beck's thesis appeared less applicable to this setting. His distinction between 'old', 'natural', versus 'new', 'manufactured' risks does not make much sense in the context of Jakarta's flood risk. The old and the new, the natural and the man-made are interwoven with one another. While Beck's earlier work paid relatively little attention to the power inequalities within society that impact the public perception of risk (claiming that risk is no longer a matter of class), the findings from my study showed that in the case of Jakarta flood risk is divided along lines of wealth and power. This is more in line with the argument of Mary Douglas than with some of the more individualist emphases of Beck. My findings indicate that risk is primarily a matter of power and a means to blame and exclude the vulnerable.

Disclosure statement

No potential conflict of interest was reported by the author.

References

Adam, B., Beck, U., & Van Loon, J. (2000). *The risk society and beyond*. Sage: London.
Alaszewski, A. (2004). Health, risk and society: Six years on. *Health, Risk & Society*, 6(1), 3–6. doi:10.1080/1369857042000193084
Anderson, A. (1997). *Media, culture and the environment*. London: University College of London Press.
Atkinson, W. (2007). Beck, individualization and the death of class: A critique. *The British Journal of Sociology*, 58(3), 349–366.
Barrett, C., Smith, K., & Box, P. W. (2001). Not necessarily in the same boat: Heterogeneous risk assessment among East African pastoralists. *The Journal of Development Studies*, 37(5), 1–30. doi:10.1080/00220380412331322101
Beck, U. (1992). *Risk society: Towards a new modernity*. London: Sage.
Beck, U. (1995). *Ecological politics in an age of risk*. Cambridge: Polity Press.
Beck, U. (2009). *World at risk*. Cambridge: Polity Press.
Beck, U. (2010). Remapping social inequalities in an age of climate change: For a cosmopolitan renewal of sociology. *Global Networks*, 10(2), 165–181. doi:10.1111/glob.2010.10.issue-2
Beck, U. (2013). Why 'class' is too soft a category to capture the explosiveness of social inequality at the beginning of the twenty-first century. *The British Journal of Sociology*, 64(1), 63–74. doi:10.1111/bjos.2013.64.issue-1

Beck, U., & Beck-Gernsheim, E. (2002). *Individualization: Institutionalized individualism and its social and political consequences.* London: Sage.

Blaikie, P., Cannon, T., Davis, I., & Wisner, B. (2004). *At risk: Natural hazards, people's vulnerability, and disasters* (2nd ed.). New York: Routledge.

Brinkman, J. (2009). *Flood hazard mapping 2. Overview main report.* Delft: DELTARES.

Caljouw, M., Nas, P. J. M., & Pratiwo, M. (2005). Flooding in Jakarta: Towards a blue city with improved water management. *Kitlv, 161*(4), 454–484.

Caplan, P. (2000). Introduction. In P. Caplan (Ed.), *Risk revisited* (pp. 1–27). London: Pluto Press.

Curran, D. (2013). Risk society and the distribution of bads: Theorizing class in the risk society. *The British Journal of Sociology, 64*(1), 44–62. doi:10.1111/bjos.2013.64.issue-1

Cybriwsky, R., & Ford, L. R. (2001). City profile: Jakarta. *Cities: The International Journal of Policy and Planning, 18*(3), 199–210. doi:10.1016/S0264-2751(01)00004-X

Dickens, P. 1992. *Who Would Know? Science, Environmental Risk and the construction of theory* (Working Paper No. 86). Sussex: Centre for Urban and Regional Research.

Douglas, M. (1966). *Purity and danger: An analysis of the concepts of pollution and taboo.* London: Ark Paperbacks.

Douglas, M. (1969). *Purity and danger: An analysis of the concepts of pollution and taboo* (2nd ed.). London: Ark Paperbacks.

Douglas, M. (1990). Risk as a forensic resource. *Mary Douglas: Daedalus, 119*(4), Risk (Fall, 1990), 1–16.

Douglas, M. (1992). *Risk and blame. Essays in cultural theory.* London: Routledge.

Douglas, M., & Wildavsky, A. (1982). *Risk and culture. An essay on the selection of technological and environmental dangers.* Berkeley: University of California Press.

Emilia, S. (2009). Discourse: Oceans, coasts. Our best assets in coping with climate change. *The Jakarta Post (Online).* Retrieved June 24, 2014, from http://www.thejakartapost.com/news/2009/12/16/discourse-oceans-coasts-our-best-assetscoping-with-climate-change.html

Furedi, F. (2002). *Culture of fear. Risk taking and the morality of low expectation.* London: Continuum.

Giddens, A. (2000). *Runaway world.* London: Routledge.

Giddens, A. (2009). *The politics of climate change.* Cambridge: Polity Press.

Goldthorpe, J. H. (2002). Globalisation and social class. *West European Politics, 25*(3), 1–28. doi:10.1080/713601612

Hajer, M., & Schwarz, M. (1997). Contouren van de risicomaatschappij. In M. Hajer & M. Schwarz (eds), *De wereld als risicomaatschappij* (pp. 7–22). Amsterdam: De Balie.

Irwin, A., Simmons, P., & Walker, G. (1999). Faulty environments and risk reasoning: The local understanding of industrial hazards. *Environment and Planning A, 31*, 1311–1326. doi:10.1068/a311311

Kadri, T. (2008). Flood defense in Bekasi City, Indonesia. Flood recovery, innovation and response. *WIT Transactions on Ecology and the Environment, 118*(1), 133–148.

Luhmann, N. (1993). *Risk: A sociological theory.* New York: A. de Gruyter.

Marfai, M. A., Yulianto, F., Hizbaron, D. R., Ward, P., & Aerts, J. (2009). *Preliminary assessment and modeling the effects of climate change on potential coastal flood damage in Jakarta.* Yogyakarta: Gadjah Mada University & VU University.

McCarthy, P. (n.d.). Urban slums reports: The case of Jakarta. *Understanding Slums: Case Studies for the Global Report on Human Settlements (online),* Retrieved December 24, 2014, from http://www.ucl.ac.uk/dpu-projects/Global_Report/pdfs/Jakarta.pdf

Michael, C. (2014, March 25). Earthquakes, hurricanes, cyclones and tsunamis: The world's 10 riskiest cities. *The Guardian.* Retrieved July 20, 2015, from http://www.theguardian.com/cities/gallery/2014/mar/25/earthquakes-hurricanes-cyclones-and-tsunamis-10-riskiest-cities-world

Mieulet, E., & Claeys, C. (2014). The implementation and reception of policies for preventing dengue fever epidemics: A comparative study of Martinique and French Guyana. *Health, Risk & Society, 16*(7–8), 581–599. doi:10.1080/13698575.2014.949224

Minuet of Life. (2013). *National Flood Day 17 January 2013.* Retrieved July 1, 2015, from http://www.minuetoflife.com/2013/01/national-flood-day-18-january-2013-free.html

Mythen, G. (2005). From goods to bads? Revisiting the political economy of risk. *Sociological Research Online, 10*(3), Retrieved from www.socresonline.org.uk/10/3/mythen.html doi:10.5153/sro.1140

Mythen, G. (2007). Reappraising the risk society thesis: Telescopic sight or myopic vision? *Current Sociology, 55*(6), 793–813. doi:10.1177/0011392107081986

Mythen, G. (2014). *Understanding the risk society. Crime, security & justice.* London: Palgrave MacMillan.

Nugent, S. (2000). Good risk, bad risk: Reflexive modernisation and Amazonia. In P. Caplan (Ed.), *Risk revisited* (pp. 226–248). London: Pluto Press.

O'Keefe, P., Westgate, K., & Wisner, B. (1976). Taking the 'naturalness' out of 'natural' disasters. *Nature, 260*(5552), 566–567. doi:10.1038/260566a0

Quinn, C. H., Huby, M., Kiwasila, H., & Lovett, J. C. (2003). Local perceptions of risk to livelihood in semi-arid Tanzania. *Journal of Environmental Management, 68*(2), 111–119. doi:10.1016/S0301-4797(03)00013-6

Sagala, S., Lassa, J., Yasaditama, H., & Hudalah, D. (2013). *The evolution of risk and vulnerability in greater Jakarta: Contesting government policy in dealing with a megacity's exposure to flooding. An academic response to Jakarta floods in January 2013* (Institute of Resource Governance and Social Change Working Paper No. 2). Retrieved June 24, 2014, from http://irgsc.org/pubs/wp/IRGSCWP002jakartaflood.pdf

Scott, J. (2002). Social class and stratification in late modernity. *Acta Sociologica, 45*(1), 23–35. doi:10.1080/00016990252885771

Tansey, J., & O'Riordan, T. (1999). Cultural theory and risk: A review. *Health, Risk & Society, 1*(1), 71–90. doi:10.1080/13698579908407008

Texier, P. (2008). Floods in Jakarta: When the extreme reveals daily structural constraints and mismanagement. *Disaster Prevention and Management, 17*(3), 358–372. doi:10.1108/09653560810887284

Van Voorst, R. (2014). *Get Ready for the Flood! Risk-handling styles in Jakarta, Indonesia.* (Thesis PhD). University of Amsterdam, Amsterdam.

Van Voorst, R. (2015). Risk-handling styles in a context of flooding and uncertainty in Jakarta, Indonesia: An analytical framework to analyse heterogenous risk-behaviour. *Disaster Prevention and Management, 24*(4), 484–505.

Van Voorst, R., & Hellman, J. (Under review). How one risk replaces the other: Floods, evictions and policies on Jakarta's river banks.

Weber, E. U., & Hsee, C. K. (2000). Culture and individual judgment and decision making. *Applied Psychology: An International Journal, 49*(1), 32–61. doi:10.1111/apps.2000.49.issue-1

Wilkinson, I. (2001). Social theories of risk perception: At once indispensable and insufficient. *Current Sociology, 49*(1), 1–22. doi:10.1177/0011392101049001002

Wisner, B., Blaikie, P., Cannon, T., & Davis, I. (2004). *At risk: Natural hazards, people's vulnerability and disasters* (2nd ed.). London: Routledge.

Wisner, B., & Caressi-Lopez, A. (2012). *Disaster management: International lessons in risk reduction, response and recovery.* London: Earthscan.

World Bank. (2011). *Resettlement policy framework (RPF). Jakarta urgent flood mitigation project (JUFMP).* Jakarta: Jakarta Capital City Government & World Bank.

Coping with health-related uncertainties and risks in Rakhine (Myanmar)

Celine Coderey

In this article, I use an anthropological perspective to investigate how uncertainty and risk related to health are understood and managed by members of the Buddhist population living in the central part of Rakhine State, in Western Myanmar (formerly known as Burma), in a context of therapeutic pluralism and of a highly lacking formal health system. Drawing on data from six fieldwork trips, which I undertook between 2005 and 2014 in the Thandwe area (Rakhine), this article examines the ways in which the multiple and unstable factors shaping villagers' health means that they lived in a permanent state of vulnerability and uncertainty. I explore how villagers responded to such uncertainty by engaging in preventive practices and when they fell sick, using more or less complex health-seeking processes to gain control of the threat at both the cognitive and practical levels. In my analysis, I note the ways in which the villagers tried different ways of dealing with the threat of illness, reflecting the plural nature of the local therapeutic system and the relationships of hierarchy and complementarity through which the components of this system are connected. I argue that Buddhism plays a key role in responses to such threats, yet, despite its dominance, it alone does not provide a way of dealing with all aspects of disease and the uncertainty related to it. Only its combination and articulation with the other components of the therapeutic system enable comprehensive action. My analysis not only shows how villagers' coping strategies were largely rooted in socio-structural factors but also reflected their social biographies as well as the social contexts in which they live.

Introduction

In this article, I use an anthropological approach to examine how uncertainty and risk related to health are understood and managed by research participants drawn from a Buddhist population living in the central part of Rakhine State, in Western Myanmar (formerly known as Burma), in a context of therapeutic pluralism and of a highly deficient formal healthcare system.

Health, risk and therapeutic pluralism

In every society, health is embedded within notions of uncertainty and risk – here understood as a situation where 'individuals are aware of the presence of danger which if not correctly or skilfully managed will probably result in harm even death' (Alaszewski

& Coxon, 2008, p. 417). However, as Douglas (2003 [1992]) has argued, the way in which social groups understand, experience and cope with this uncertainty and risk varies greatly. It depends on the aetiological and cosmological systems they embrace, the therapeutic practices they can access, as well as their biographical background and the socio-economic and political contexts (Henwood, Pidgeon, Sarre, Simmons, & Smith, 2008, p. 424; Mythen & Walklate, 2006, p.10).

Rakhine Buddhist people apprehend and manage health and disease through a multiplicity of conceptions and practices originating from different traditions: indigenous medicine (*taing-yin hsay pyinnya*, 'knowledge of indigenous remedies'); Western biomedicine (*ingaleik hsay pyinnya*, 'knowledge of the English [and by implication Western] remedies'), formally introduced in the country by the British colonisers; Theravada Buddhism; divination; astrology; alchemy and spirits cults (Coderey, 2011).

Only two of these systems are officially recognised and endorsed: Western medicine and a modernised and standardised version of indigenous medicine promoted by the Burmese military government since the post-independence period. However, such an endorsement has not been matched by substantial investment in services, with the result that health services lack medicines, staff and equipment (Coderey, 2011; Skidmore, 2008). These weaknesses are the result of many years of underinvestment and neglect on the part of the state and international actors (Finch & Win, 2013). These deficiencies are particularly evident in Rakhine and in other peripheral areas historically neglected by the Burmese central government. Although the semi-civil government, which took over from the military junta in 2011, initiated some reforms in the health system in order to increase the quality and the accessibility of the services, concrete outcomes are not yet visible, especially in peripheral areas.

Alongside the 'official' Western and indigenous healthcare systems, Buddhism, astrology, spirits cults and so on, represent more accessible avenues to manage health problems. Moreover, in contrast to medical traditions, these systems do not focus solely on the physiological aspects of ill health but consider also aspects neglected by the formal medical system such as the spiritual, the social and the cosmological (Eisenbruch; 1992; Golomb, 1988; Pottier, 2007). They do not deal with ill health as a distinctive special area of human experience but include it within the larger category of misfortune, hence connecting it to questions of destiny, fate and agency.

In everyday life, these different traditions are highly entangled, often even melded within the same practice. Yet they always remain subordinate to Buddhism, which acts as the encompassing force determining the value and efficacy of action of the other components. The entanglement between Buddhist and para-Buddhist traditions and the implication of Buddhism in worldly matters observed in people's daily reality have long been at the core of reflections by religious scholars in Myanmar and in other Theravada Buddhist countries (Ames 1964; Obeyesekere, 1963; Spiro, 1971), because they clashed with the notion traditionally held by Buddhologists, who considered Buddhism as a pure tradition turned towards other-worldly aims. Only more recently there has been recognition (see Gellner, 1990; Hayashi, 2003; Swearer, 1995) that alongside the theological dimension of Buddhism, it has, since its origins, functioned as a way of dealing with problems encountered in everyday life.

My main argument in this work is that this plurality of traditions is interwoven with uncertainty (*ma te bu*) and risk (*andaye*, word referring at the same time to the risk, as a condition of danger, and to the danger or dangerous factor itself), both in their aetiologies and in their practices. The practices are not only a way of minimising uncertainty and risk but also, in some circumstances, a source of uncertainty and risk. Moreover, uncertainty and risk represent a key to appreciating the relationship between these different approaches and understanding how they complement each other. I aim indeed to show, as a second aspect, that these aetiologies and practices are related through complementary yet hierarchical functions regarding the apprehension of disease and the uncertainty and risk related to it and also that the paramedical approaches largely compensate for the various deficiencies of the medical ones. Finally, I aim to show that individuals' responses to the threat of illness do not exist in a social vacuum but are shaped by the social and economic reality in which they live and by their personal biographies.

Methodology

The data I use in this article is derived from six fieldwork trips, of 14 months' duration in total, which I conducted between 2005 and 2014 in the Thandwe area, in the central part of Rakhine State. I focused my research on the fishing villages of Lintha, Watankwai, Myabin, Giaiktaw and Lontha. This fieldwork is particularly relevant for the topic treated in this article, because it was focused on the plurality of local conceptions and practices related to health and ill health. My study represents an important contribution to the anthropological literature given that this topic has never been explored in its complexity either for Rakhine or for Myanmar.

Setting for the fieldwork

Thandwe city hosted a mixed ethnic population with substantial Muslim communities. However, in the rural areas and coastal villages, most of the population was Buddhist. Most of the villagers were farmers or fishermen, though there was also some employment in trading, the food industry and hotels. In terms of healthcare, the Thandwe area was provided with a public hospital of Western medicine located in Thandwe city and, under it, a network of rural health centres located in the surrounding villages. The private sector was represented by services started by professionals who also worked in the public service, most of which were based in Thandwe city; Lintha and Watankwai did not have any such services, while Myabin had one and Giaiktaw had two. Myabin also hosted a clinic opened by the French NGO Association Médicale France-Asie (AMFA). For indigenous medicine – in its modernised and institutionalised version – there was only one public and three private clinics, all based in Thandwe city.

All these services were under-resourced, lacking in staff, equipment and medicine and they were able to provide only very basic services. However, the towns and villages were well supplied with other experts such as Buddhist monks, diviners, astrologers, spirit mediums, who were willing and able to offer services for those experiencing misfortune, including ill health, as well as specialists in traditional indigenous medicine, although these healers were finding it difficult to compete with government-approved practitioners. Thus, the inhabitants of the four villages I studied could access government-approved services especially if they were willing and able to travel to Thandwe city, but they also had easy access to a range of local experts, making this an interesting location in which to study how and why villagers used different experts and expertise to address the threat of ill health.

I focused on one relatively small area, as it enabled me over time to build a relationship of confidence and trust with the local population so that I could obtain reliable and detailed data. This is all the more important given the topic and the political context of this research. Health belongs to the private or even intimate sphere and people are not necessarily willing to share their health-related thoughts and experiences with strangers. Moreover, developing a closer relationship prevented (within certain limits) people from disguising conceptions and practices often considered as superstitions or primitive by the Western world and trying to give what they believed was a more respectable image of themselves. Trust was particularly hard to acquire due to the climate of suspicion and mistrust generated by the military dictatorship. In a context where words, actions and movements are controlled, people are not at ease with someone coming into their house, asking questions and making notes.

Ethnography

In my ethnography, I sought to access and triangulate data from a variety of participants and sources. I worked with villagers (40 households composed of between one and seven individuals), and among 75 individuals who provided villagers with health services, approximately a half (37) used non-Western expertise, including eight monks, five exorcists, two monks-exorcists, three specialists of indigenous medicine, six specialists of indigenous medicine-exorcists, three spirit mediums, five astrologers, five diviners, and the rest (38) used Western expertise: 15 biomedical doctors, six nurses, five midwives, two health assistants and 10 drug sellers.

I built up my contact with villagers through social networking, mainly on the basis of casual encounters on the street, in shops, tea shops, etc. Often, while out walking, a villager sitting on a veranda would greet me and, after we had talked for a bit, would invite me into the household. Over time, I concentrated on working with a group of 40 families who were keen to participate in my study and wanted to share their experiences with me. On occasion, members of these families would introduce me to villagers who they felt had a special experience that might be relevant to my research, for instance, people who had suffered or were suffering from certain diseases. I sought to maintain regular social contact with all these families, but seven families chose to involve me more closely in their daily life, for example, they would invite me to accompany them when they consulted a specialist.

Most of the experts who participated in my study lived in my study villages and provided services to the villagers. I did also include experts who lived outside the villages but were particularly popular in the area plus medical specialists based in Thandwe city. Although I met all of the experts several times, I was able to build up a closer relationship only with 20 who let me visit regularly, engaged in longer conversations of up to 3 hours and let me 'sit in' on their consultations.

Most of the time, I talked to and/or observed people in their ordinary everyday settings. For example, I talked to villagers and experts in their homes, and monks in the main hall of their monastery. On some occasions, I had discussions with doctors and nurses in their work place but, given the formal ban on foreigners in government healthcare facilities, I sometimes had to talk with them in their own homes or public spaces such as tea rooms. With both villagers and experts, I combined informal conversations with semi-structured interviews about health and healing. I asked villagers how they defined ill health, what they thought the causes were, what actions they took to avert the threat of ill health and what actions they took when they were ill. I asked experts why they had decided to become experts, how they acquired their expertise, how they identified and cured a health problem.

In addition to conversations and interviews, I also observed how individuals dealt with health issues. In the villagers' houses, I observed and recorded everyday activities, especially those related to promoting health or treating ill health, for example, I observed how villagers used medicines, amulets, altars and shrines. In the experts' work settings, I focused on the way they interacted with individuals who consulted them as well as on the equipment they used. I also observed local events that could be related to an under-standing and management of the threat of ill health, including pagoda festivals and other religious celebrations.

Although I acquired skill in the local language, to ensure that I did not misunderstand or misinterpret, I used a local assistant fluent in English to participate in most interviews. When I anticipated that an interview would be long, more formal or involving many technical terms (notably when the interviewee was a monk, an astrologer or a specialist of indigenous medicine), I audio-recorded it. As soon as possible after the interview, I transcribed the recording into English and created a text file on my laptop. I entered information from shorter, less formal interviews and with observations into my field note book and created a fuller computer-based text account of these. When possible, I also used audiovisual equipment to record events.

Findings

I have structured my findings around three distinct but interrelated features of healthcare practices pertaining to risk – the underlying understandings of aetiologies of illness, the practices taken to prevent or reduce the risk of illness and health-seeking practices undertaken once ill.

The local aetiological system

The participants in my study considered illness, locally called *yawga*, as the product of a disorder within the body or with the outside world, which created an imbalance of the body elements – air, fire, earth and water. Although these elements were seen as intrinsically unstable (*ma te*, 'not stable'), their instability was aggravated during specific periods in life such as childhood, old age, menstruation, pregnancy, delivery and meno-pause. During these phases, my participants felt that people were particularly vulnerable to diseases (*yawga win lwe de*, 'disease enters easily'). Moreover, the imbalance and hence the state of vulnerability could be the result of a number of factors:

- *Kan*, karma, or action. My informants attributed to this word two meanings: the everyday movements and state of the human body such as sitting, lying down, walking; and a more Buddhist meaning grounded in moral judgement of human actions. In this sense, actions can be meritorious (*kutho*) and demeritorious (*akutho*). An action is judged meritorious if it conforms to Buddhist morality, as represented by the five main Buddhist principles (not killing, lying or stealing, and abstaining from alcohol and sexual misconduct); making charitable gifts; and meditating. Actions are demeritorious deeds if they conflict with Buddhist morality or show disrespect for the Buddha, his monks, an individual's parents or teachers. An individual's actions and the balance between their merits and demerits across their life course determine their life after their death and rebirth in terms of their gender, socio-economic circumstances, health, life span and therefore propensity and vulnerability to ill health. In addition, some particular actions will also bring about direct reward/punishment in the next life, for instance, in the form of specific illnesses. Karmic retribution was often said to be an automatic and inevitable process, and participants in my study agreed that sometimes it did not occur or occurred in a moderated way, the reason being that, villagers explained, meritorious and demeritorious deeds could neutralise each other – within certain limits.

- *Gyo*, the planetary influence. Villagers recognised the importance of astrology and noted that the planetary configuration at the moment of a person's birth influenced his or her life and well-being. Astrologers in Rakhine, as in India (Guenzi, 2004; Pugh, 1983), consider that the planetary influence is determined by karma: the place and time of an individual's birth and therefore their astrological chart are determined by their past karma. As U Thun Kaing, an astrologer from Giaiktaw, stated: 'meritorious and demeritorious actions accomplished in the past life will bear consequences in tune with the sequence of positive and negative planetary influences active in this current life'.
- *Hpon*, refers to a spiritual, psychical and physical essence that bestowed upon a person not only moral, spiritual and intellectual superiority, but also strength, integrity and resistance and, for men, virility. Villagers deemed it to be a source of popularity, success, wealth and health and saw it as protecting an individual from danger and supernatural aggressions. The amount of *hpon* a person possesses depends on the status of his or her karma. Men have more power than women. *Hpon* can be reduced through contact with a 'polluting' object (menstrual blood or even, by extension, a woman's skirt) or a place (a funeral house or delivery room). For men, this loss is more dangerous than for women, as the gravity of the loss is linked to the amount of *hpon* an individual possesses.
- *Ahara*, food. The villagers considered that ill health could be caused by eating unsuitable food. The suitability and unsuitability of food relates to villagers' judgements of their hot or cold nature, which is partly determined by taste but also relates to the hot or cold nature of the person and the season.
- *Utu*, the climate and the seasonal changes. My informants told me that when the weather was particularly hot or cold as well as during the transitional phases from one season to the other, people easily fell ill.
- *Seik*, the mind or, more precisely, an event upsetting a person's mental stability.
- *Payawga*, disturbances or troubles caused by vindictive and malevolent beings. Such beings belong to three categories: witches who harm people by giving them bewitched food or by uttering spells on their belongings; sorcerers who harm their victims either using spirits or by burying in the compound of the victim's house papers or metal sheets inscribed with esoteric scripts; and tutelary spirits (*nat*) or errant spirits (*thasay, thaye, peikta*), who trouble human beings as revenge for being neglected or offended, or because they are hungry.

Villagers and specialists considered that these seven causal factors can act singly or in combination. In particular, a person's karma and planetary conditions often acted as determiners for the other factors. As U Tun Khaing, a traditional healer from Giaiktaw, explained:

> A positive karma and a positive planetary influence act as a protective barrier while a negative karma and a negative planetary influence allow the other factors to harm the person.

Villagers paid particular attention to ill health generated by bad karma and considered it a specific category of disease which corresponded to a form of misfortune like other unpleasant events resulting from negative karma such as a car accident or a poor crop.

In all these cases, they spoke of *kan ma kaung bu*, 'to have bad karma'. Although several factors could contribute to a misfortune event, karma was seen as the most influential.

An important element of villagers' understanding of ill health was that it doesn't include Western biomedical concepts. Indeed, such concepts were unknown to the majority and largely remained the prerogative of biomedical specialists. This absence was, as I will discuss further, a product of the cultural distance separating the traditional and the biomedical conceptions and the numerous barriers – that I will examine below – that hinder communication between ordinary villagers and medical practitioners.

Uncertainty, instability and unpredictability of local aetiologies

According to local conceptions, causal factors of diseases were everywhere – in the body and the environment – continually threatening to disturb the individual. They thus represented a source of danger, of potential risk (*andaye*). This was all the more so as these factors were unstable (*ma te*) and unpredictable (*ma khan hman/twet*, 'that cannot be estimated/calculated'). Indeed, in line with the Buddhist idea that everything is impermanent (Pāli *thinkhaya*), karma could turn from positive to negative at any moment; the four body elements were in a state of constant flux; and social relations were unstable as people's minds could change from benevolent to malevolent depending on the circumstances. In addition, as most factors are invisible, it was difficult to track their status and to estimate to what extent they represented a threat for one's health. The uncertainty concerning karma was particularly significant given that karma determined the weight of the impact of other factors. Hence, villagers lived in a chronic condition of uncertainty concerning their vulnerability.

Despite this, people did not feel permanently at risk, nor did they live with an unabated sense of danger and anxiety. If the local cosmology filled people's lives with risks, it also provided various tools to contain risks. People constantly engaged in practices and rituals aimed at increasing their karma and maintaining the order within the body and with the cosmos, hence saving themselves from the harmful consequences of disorder. Put differently, they tried permanently to increase their stock of fortune. Fortune was perceived as positive capital or benevolent power that caused favourable things to happen to someone. In the same way as misfortune was determined mainly – but not exclusively – by karma, so it was for fortune. Fortune largely depended on one's karma (hence the expression *kan kaung de*, 'to have a good karma' used to speak about fortune) but it was also the consequence of other actions such as wearing amulets, adapting actions addressed to the planetary influence and choosing the auspicious (*mingala*) time to perform something important. These practices provided a certain sense of control and safety. However, people were aware that if they did not perform certain actions and respect certain rules, they ran a risk of encountering problems. Moreover, villagers knew that the control they could exercise on causal factors had its limits and that these limits were dictated by their karma. Indeed, as U Thun, an old man from Lintha explained to me:

> preventive practices are effective only if the events they are intended to avoid are not the consequence of a particularly bad act the person has accomplished in one of his lives. Actions such as killing sentient beings, offending the Buddha or parents are considered particularly serious and their punishment can't be avoided. (...) The efficacy of these practices is guaranteed only if, in the current life, the person behaves according to the Buddhist morality.

Yet, because of the impossibility of knowing the exact state of one's karma, and because of the idea that the karma that accumulates in the present life is deemed to bring fruits and could, to a certain extent, counterbalance the past-life bad karma, there was always space for hope and hence for action.

Nevertheless, it cannot be said that people never experienced fear. They did, but this fear mostly concerned factors over which they had little or no control, because these factors were external, unpredictable and invisible. In particular, villagers often expressed their fear of supernatural aggressions. And this was the case for individuals belonging to every socio-economical class and of all educational backgrounds.

Dealing with the risk of disease: preventive practices

Villagers seldom spoke about preventing ill health per se, rather they saw prevention as a side effect of the actions they took to preserve the individual and cosmic order and build up a stock of fortune, enabling them to maintain individual and societal well-being. These practices were carried out on a regular basis, a sign of the instability of the order but also a sign that fortune could only be obtained through an attentive and continual effort. However, people's engagement in these practices varied according to their perception of the dangers, their personal beliefs and family traditions, their educational level and their ability to act, which were largely affected by their structural position in society.

Buddhist devotions

For most villagers, the day started and ended with Buddhist devotions undertaken at the household Buddha's altar. During the day, such devotions could be repeated during visits to pagodas and temples. They were mainly addressed to the Buddha, but also to deities of the Hindu-Buddhist pantheon and the *weikza* – humans who have acquired supernatural powers by combining meditation and esoteric practices, notably alchemy and esoteric inscriptions. The devotions included offerings of water, food, candles and incense; the recitation of formulae of homage, protective formulae and prayers; and, for some, meditation. The villagers said that these acts increased their karma and personal power and attracted the help and the protection of superior beings. Depending on the household, these devotions were undertaken by one or more persons. If it was a single person, then it was generally the household's matriarch who, according to local custom, bore the responsibility of the family's well-being. By undertaking this activity, she could increase her own karma and hence the chance of being reborn as a man in the next life.

Another important Buddhist practice conducted on a regular basis was the recitation by monks of Buddha's discourses, intended to provide auspiciousness and protection or release from troubles. The benefits of such recitations took various forms: villagers considered that listening to the chants not only created merit but also provided peace of mind, calmness and stability, which could prevent diseases and aggressions. As the abbot of Myabin stated: 'a pure and strong mind can't be frightened nor subject to aggression'. Villagers and monks noted also that chanting contributed to villagers' well-being through imparting sacred power to different objects such as pots of sand, water and threads, which were then used as protective barriers when worn or kept in the household.

Respecting social order and conventions

Villagers also considered that respecting social norms contributed to preserving societal order and protecting individuals' health. These norms were based on the five main Buddhist precepts but also included social conventions about bodily gestures, positions and movements based on age and gender. Villagers described how respecting these norms and conventions increased a person's karma and personal power while going against them exposed the person to the risk of misfortune. If an individual breached the conventions based on gender, then both parties would be affected and the consequences could be severe. For example, a man disrespected by a woman could see his power weakened and find himself subordinated to his wife and children, as well as to other men, and be exposed to the danger of all kinds of misfortunes. The woman responsible for this violation has also committed a sin and moral transgression, which will reduce her karma and *hpon*; people referred to this as '*ngaye kya de*' (she falls into hell).

There were a set of rules that limited women's power. If in private women have authority (*ana*), in public they must behave in a modest and humble way and avoid showing their superiority. A woman should refrain from sleeping, walking, eating or moving on the right side of the man and, in particular, sleeping with her head on his right shoulder, because that is where his power is located. She should also avoid being in a higher spot than men, where her vagina will be in a higher position than the level of the man's head. Men and women's clothes should be washed and hung separately, with women's in a lower position to prevent men from walking under them. Finally, men should avoid washing women's clothes. People in my study took these norms and conventions seriously. For example, I talked to Min Soe, a young migrant male worker from the Rakhine island of Ma Aung, who worked in a hotel in Myabin, and he told me that:

> sometimes I feel like crying when working in the hotel rooms, as I am forced to walk under the clothes that the tourists hang out to dry.

However, these rules were increasingly questioned, especially by the younger generation who have been exposed to Western culture. Kay Thi, a young woman in her twenties, noted that:

> these are old traditions we don't follow anymore. People see tourists here and watch [Korean and American] movies ... even in the movies you see a boy carrying her girlfriend on his shoulders ... so? Nothing happens.

Respect of the supernatural and preventive action

Villagers were aware of the power of spirits (*nat*), who watch over places people frequent in their daily lives, including the house, the sea and the fields. They felt it was important to regularly offer these spirits food, as this would prevent the spirits from harming them and causing illness. The villagers also believe that it made sense to engage in actions that reduced their exposure to potential harm; *andaye kin*, 'prevention from dangers'. Such sensible precautions included: not carrying around uncovered food; uttering Buddhist protective formulae to pacify spirits and reinforcing one's personal power when crossing haunted places, and not accepting food from anyone other than kin and friends.

Dietary rules

Most villagers were careful to preserve the balance between the four main elements and between hot and cold, by following dietary rules related to the hot or cold nature of the food. As La Myin, a young woman from Myabin explained to me:

> Everyone should avoid eating extremely cold or extremely hot food, or combining extremely hot and extremely cold ingredients.

Divination

People consulted diviners once or twice a year, generally on their birthdays, New Year and special events such as births, weddings, travels or the starting of a new business. In contrast with other practices, which are performed without knowing one's state of vulnerability, divination is aimed at foreseeing the future and acting on that basis. In the region, the two most popular divinatory practices were astrology and communication with the *weikza* (Coderey, 2011). Through the recitation of formulae, diviners enter into mental contact with the *weikza*, powerful beings who give the diviners the power to see and hear things invisible and inaudible to other people. Through these techniques, diviners can read a person's astrological chart and hence the fortune and misfortune reserved for him/her, and offer strategies that will take advantage of positive moments and prevent negative ones.

The main technique for shaping one's destiny was the prescription of *yadaya*, offerings to the pagoda chosen according to astrological calculations, in order to boost karma and, if necessary, to avert the planetary influence. As Ma Su, a female villager explained to me:

> It's like filling the glass with water. You must make sure that your glass is always full, or at least not empty, so you need to fill it up regularly by consulting an astrologer and doing some *yadaya*.

As a way to enhance their fortune, villagers also wore amulets provided to them by experts. Amulets are composed by rolling around a thread paper or metal sheets inscribed with *in* or *sama*, letters and numbers referring to Buddhist and astrological concepts. These are then worn as necklets or bracelets. Villagers saw these amulets as providing them a protection against the negative karma yet they acknowledged that this protection was limited as it relied on an external and temporary power.

Most of the villagers engaged in these practices as they felt they provided them with a sense of control and protection. Divination was particularly popular among women. Not only were women said to believe in and trust diviners more than men, they were also deemed to be responsible for the family well-being. Hence, they often consulted diviners not only for themselves but also on behalf of other family members.

There were occasions when the risk of disease was seen as being higher and more concrete because one or more factors are or are likely to go out of balance. For instance, during childhood and the postpartum period, the karmic and planetary situation are adverse and some specific dangers are predicted. People were aware of their vulnerability and often experienced a certain degree of anxiety because they knew what they would likely face if they were unable to contain the danger. In these cases, people resorted to short-term protection focused on their factors of vulnerability. They might recite protective formulae, wear amulets, accomplish *yadaya*, avoid specific foods and take other similar preventative approaches. These acts were performed with a specific preventive aim and were recognised solely for this function.

The limited use of biomedical preventive practices

Villagers seldom spontaneously used preventive practices grounded in biomedicine and hardly mentioned them in their conversations and interviews about vulnerability and risk of diseases. For villagers in Rakhine, the notion of prevention as promoted by biomedical science, with its focus on the physical body and specific diseases, seemed quite alien. For the villagers, there were various cultural, social and political factors that made it difficult to accept these practices. The difficulties could be clearly seen in the case of free vaccinations offered by all public health centres as part of the Universal Children Immunization (UCI) programme. In the villages, many mothers refused to participate in the programme. These women feared that the injections would harm their children. Thi Da, a 38-year-old villager and mother from Lintha, told me that many mothers didn't want:

> to harm their children and make them cry with that injection. They [mothers] also greatly fear the side-effects of the vaccines, mainly the fever provoked by the DPT [diphtheria, tetanus, pertussis] vaccine.

Villagers felt that Western-trained experts who ran such services didn't treat them with respect. According to the villagers, the nurses rarely went looking for people who had not come forward for vaccination and, if they did, they scolded them. Such attitudes have increased the resistance against vaccinations and reinforced people's mistrust of public health programmes.

The complementary and hierarchical role of preventive practices

For the villagers, karma was central to an individual's future and their experience of fortune and misfortune. Villagers described the ways in which boosting a person's own positive karma was the most fundamental protective action that an individual could take, as karma acted as a filter for the other influences and determined the scope of the preventive effect. For the villagers, a good karma provided personal, wide-ranging and long-term protection against misfortune. Therefore, the villagers stated that Buddhist practices were crucial to ensure good fortune and good health and when asked how individuals should protect themselves from diseases and misfortune, most of them advocated 'following the Buddha's way' and conforming to Buddhist law and principles.

However, individuals could not be certain about their karma as it depended both on their actions in past lives and on their actions in the present life. The belief that planets mirror karma allows astrology to fill this gap in knowledge and to determine concrete strategies to improve an individual's life and prevent misfortune. This was done not only through practices that improve a person's karma, power and the planetary condition, but also through practices that address other potential dangers.

Although karma and planetary influence occupied a central role in the prevention process, people paid a lot of attention to the other factors as well. This is because these factors can act independently from the karma and, even when filtered by the karma, their impact can still be significant. As U Tun Khaing, a traditional healer from Giaiktaw, told me:

although my karma is temporarily favourable, I can anyway be negatively affected by the
weather conditions or the food I eat but of course not as seriously as if my karma was bad.
So, I need to be attentive.

Similarly, Ma Than Gyi, a shopkeeper from Myabin, commented to me: 'We have a
saying that if you just rely on your [positive] karma you will sit on a pin and be pricked by
it'. All these factors, which exist beside the karma, were mainly addressed through
specific practices (offerings to spirits, respect of dietary rules), rather than through
Buddhism, which is more abstract and generic.

Having discussed the ways in which villagers tried to prevent ill health and misfortune, I will now consider the ways in which they responded when illness and misfortune
actually happened.

Responding to disease: uncertainty in the curing process

For the villagers, disease was by definition a condition of uncertainty, regarding causes,
appropriate treatment and the chances of recovery. An ill villager would, with his/her
relatives, make a hypothesis about the meaning and causes of the disease and decide
which practices and healers to turn to in order to restore a state of well-being. This
health-seeking process was different for every person and episode of disease. It was
largely determined by the way those involved interpreted the nature and gravity of
the disease, the accessibility of different methods and their structural position within
the society and the level of trust in the different alternatives. Across this heterogeneity,
it is nevertheless possible to identify some general trends, which I outline through a
case study.

Case study: Aye Aye

Aye Aye was a 32-year-old woman living in Linthar. One day, she experienced
severe abdominal pain. After a week when she still had the pain, Aye Aye decided to
go to Thandwe City Hospital with her family. At the hospital, the doctors examined
her, diagnosed indigestion, prescribed medicines and advised her to eat only rice
soup. A few days passed but Aye Aye did not get better and she started wondering if
her sickness was a 'normal', 'ordinary' (yo yo) sickness. She remembered that one
month ago, after having urinated under a tree in her garden, she had had a dream
about a huge ugly figure, which she thought was a bad spirit, standing behind her.
The day after her dream, she started having abdominal pains and breathing difficulties. When she heard Aye Aye's account, her older sister, Cho Cho, decided to
consult the village monk. The monk investigated Aye Aye by calculating her horoscope and found that her karma and the planets' alignment were not favourable. He
advised her family to make an offering of rice and water near the street in front of
their house. Although Aye Aye's mother made the prescribed offering, Aye Aye's
symptoms persisted. Four days later, Aye Aye and her younger sister consulted Ma
Shan Aye, a famous divination master living in Giaiktaw. Ma Shan Aye made further
astrological calculations using her own protocol, then used her special powers to
consult the weikza, powerful supernatural beings, in order to gain insight into the
cause of Aye Aye's misfortune. Ma Shan Aye found that Aye Aye's karma and the
planetary alignment were unfavourable and she had been tormented by a spirit for
over two weeks. Ma Shan Aye also found that the spirit wanted an offering of eggs,

rice and meat near the house. Ma Shan Aye gave Aye Aye some consecrated candles, incense sticks and bottles of water and advised her to meditate every morning at five o'clock.

Following her consultation with Ma Shan Aye, Aye Aye returned home but that afternoon, the spirit possessed her twice. During her possession, Aye Aye shouted, cried, opened her clothes revealing her breasts and she kicked her sister. The noise attracted women from neighbouring houses, who came running to see what was happening and to offer their help. Aye Aye's sister and the neighbours decided that the spirit needed to be exorcised so they gave Aye Aye an *awza* leaf (*Annona squamosa*) to smell. The villagers believed that the leaf would chase away the spirit as the shape of its fruit is said to be similar to the face of an ogre, a frightening figure and its name: *awza* meant 'authority', that is what was needed to chase away the malevolent beings. In the evening, Aye Aye's sister went outside to make the prescribed offering, then came back to sprinkle some consecrated water on Aye Aye, and all those involved agreed the spirit had left Aye Aye.

The following day, Aye Aye said that she felt better but experienced weakness, further pains in her abdomen and heavy-headedness. She carried on with a light diet and continued to take both Western and indigenous medications. As she was not getting better, Aye Aye developed a new explanation for her misfortune. She remembered that a few weeks previously, a woman had given her a fruit that had been a gift from a neighbour. After eating the fruit, she had vomited. She now suspected that the neighbour was a witch who had wanted to harm her. Aye Aye's family discussed this new explanation and agreed to consult an exorcist recommended by a friend of Aye Aye's older sister. The expert lived in Teiodo, a small village near Thandwe city, an hour's bus journey away.

When Aye Aye and her sisters reached the exorcist's house, they told him about Aye Aye's misfortune, especially her stomach problems. The exorcist then invoked the help of the Buddha and of the *weikza*, and he investigated Aye Aye's horoscope. He confirmed that Aye Aye was attacked by a witch. By feeling Aye Aye's abdomen, he found that the witch had used food to attack Aye Aye. He then talked to the witch inside Aye Aye's body and ordered her to bow three times to the Buddha and then three times to him. He then asked the witch repeatedly why and how she had attacked Aye Aye. After a time, the witch answered saying that she did it through a fruit because she hated Aye Aye. The exorcist forced the witch to promise never to attack Aye Aye again and ordered her to go away. Then he gave Aye Aye consecrated water to drink and a protective silver sheet inscribed with esoteric symbols. Over the days following the exorcism Aye Aye recovered and felt better.

In the case of Aye Aye, as much as in most of the cases, symptoms were ambiguous and could suggest a natural or a supernatural cause. Nevertheless, they were generally first understood as 'normal' (*yo yo*) and treated as such, that is, by turning to indigenous or Western medicine in the form of self-medication or recourse to specialists. The eventual hypothesis of karmic, planetary or supernatural implications, and hence the recourse to practitioners and methods relative to misfortune emerged only when medical methods failed.

Comment

If ailments were perceived as common, not serious and chronic, or if people could not afford to seek specialists, they relied on homemade remedies or drugs sold in shops. If the problem persisted and technical skills or instruments were called for, those who could afford it resorted to specialists, often biomedical practitioners. However, several factors hindered accessibility to these specialists and the quality of their services was questionable. All local services, including the hospital, were extremely limited and provided only minor treatments. They were also expensive; this was true for public services as well even though these were supposed to provide mostly free treatment. Moreover, public services were badly run and staff were said to be negligent and attending to patients based on their socio-economic status. Private services were generally considered a better option, because medicines were available and doctors were said to take much better care of patients regardless of their economic status, although a shop owner from Lintha articulated a widely held view when he told me that 'they don't do it from the kindness of their heart but because they are paid for the service and the money goes directly into their pocket'. Although most villagers said they preferred these services to the public ones, not everyone could afford them.

As the case of Aye Aye shows, when recourse to Western and/or indigenous medicine failed, the hypothesis of an implication of karma, the planets or supernatural factors emerged, hence, the recourse to practices and specialists of misfortune: divinatory techniques to establish the nature of the disease, amulets to provide an external power and exorcist rituals to chase evil away. Depending on the situation, the health-seeking process could be very complex. This process was driven by the need to cognitively and practically gain control over the situation and to master the uncertainty. A certain anxiety was discernable in the ways in which my research participants often seemed very impatient in their quest for treatment. They seldom waited long enough to see if a treatment was effective; if it did not yield visible results quickly, they then tried something else. Yet, their anxiety was eased generally through the certain hope of recovery. This hope was strictly related to the plurality of resorts available, sanctioning the idea that sooner or later one would find the good solution.

In the event that the disease turned out to be incurable or the person died, this was attributed to karma, which provided meaning and consolation, while also confirming the encompassing and dominant role of Buddhism. If and when an individual recovered, the process continued in that although a certain balance had been re-established, it was considered to be very fragile and needed to be maintained. Hence, the auspicious-preventive practices that an individual engaged in before the disease episode might continue long after the symptoms have disappeared.

When coping with uncertainty and risk generates further uncertainty and risk

Villagers recognised that some of the practices they used to deal with the threat of illness and misfortune may instead prevent them from recovering or harming them even further. Such a threat may be inherent to the chosen response or may arise from the ways in which the approach is used. I will use two examples, one relating to the use of indigenous specialists and one to medical products, to show that these threats were not always perceived by all the participants and that an acknowledgement of the inherent danger did not necessarily lead to risk-avoiding practices. As I will show, trust played an important part in coping with the perceived threats.

Among the different specialists, those giving rise to most concern are exorcists. Indeed, villagers saw exorcists as ambiguous and potentially dangerous figures. This stemmed from exorcists' dealing with the supernatural and occult forces and that the power they handle is neutral; it could be used for good or bad ends. Masters who explicitly followed the Buddha's way, respected Buddhist precepts, practised meditation and showed kindness towards the patient were seen as more reliable. As a result, people resorted to exorcists only in extreme cases and always with a certain awe and fear. They would consult a master whom they had already met and with whom they felt confident, or one recommended by a relative or a friend, as in Aye Aye's case.

Other risks commonly mentioned by my informants were those related to Western pharmaceuticals. In contrast to indigenous medicine, which was considered harmless because of its natural and local character, and because of its familiarity, Western products were seen as not only much more powerful but also dangerous and quite mysterious. Villagers' perceptions appeared to be shaped by the synthetic-chemical nature of these products and their foreign origin, which was emphasised by the English-language information leaflets that accompanied many products. All villagers, regardless of their socio-economic and educational level, stressed their fear of the side-effects of these drugs and stated that they should be taken sparingly because of their dangerous nature. They also feared that taking these medicines engendered a certain dependence.

Villagers used different strategies to cope with these dangers. Some simply avoided using these medicines altogether or used them only when absolutely necessary. The majority of villagers only bought products they were familiar with or that had been recommended by a specialist or relatives, or which were widely advertised in the media. Cho Cho, a long-time sufferer of gastritis from Watankwai, consulted doctors at the AMFA clinic in Myabin. The medicines prescribed for her were very effective, but when she went back for the same problem, she was worried about the medicines prescribed, as she was not sure that they were the same. She examined their shape and colour carefully, even smelling them in order to make sure they were identical.

Discussion

Masters of their own destiny?

In my study, I found that Rakhine villagers saw illness and misfortune as being tightly connected to an individual's natural, supernatural and social environment. Moreover, they considered their state of health and well-being as depending on the state – of balance or imbalance – of this relationship. Such findings are very much in line with ethnographic research from other Asian settings (see, for example, Augé, 1984; Benoist, 1996; Eisenbruch, 1992; Laderman & Van Esterik, 1988, Pottier, 2007). However, my fieldwork showed how much these conceptions were imbued with a sense of risk and uncertainty. Indeed, the multiplicity of factors at stake and their inherent instability and unpredictability meant that people were living in a constant uncertainty and vulnerability.

While villagers were aware of the fragility of health and life and the ever-present threat of danger, for example, from eating the wrong food or from spirits, they did not live with an unabated sense of danger and anxiety. As Alaszewski and Coxon (2008, p. 417) have argued, a threat or a risk is always judged in terms of an action – of risk-taking or risk-avoiding. For villagers, the local pluralistic therapeutic system was pervaded by understandings of uncertainty and risk as well as other related notions such as vulnerability, instability and danger. Yet, this pluralism also provided ways in which villagers could cope and thus enhance hope of health or recovery. But where did the belief – and the hope – that their action could be effective come from? In contrast to many communities which hold that people's fortune and misfortune are determined by fate or by gods' will (Da Col, 2012), and which thus are likely to develop a fatalistic and passive attitude, Rakhine villagers believed that their destiny lay in their own hands, as consequences of their own actions in the world. And even though, in principle, they recognised that people had to face the unpleasant consequences of their demeritorious deeds, they also believed that good deeds could balance and hence neutralise bad deeds and hence even release the person from karmic retributions. The conception of karma as a balance and the idea that the karmic retribution can be avoided are, many authors have argued, a post hoc development in the history of karma. Indeed, Rosu (1978, p. 126), Chenet (1985, pp. 115–119), Spiro (1971, p. 142) consider that the original conception of karma was that of a 'strong' karma, whose retribution was automatic and unavoidable. They affirm that the idea of a 'soft' karma, whose retribution can be avoided, was introduced later in order to justify other practices (notably medicine and astrology) and to give value to human initiative in the shaping of an individual's destiny.

Exceptions exist to this general conception of karma as balance, but these are counterbalanced by the idea that all retributions can be avoided, except those which are the consequences of particularly demeritorious acts. Karma is thus not only the origin but also the limit of one's destiny (Gombrich, 1971). Given that the participants in my study could not know exactly what they had done in their previous lives, nor could they be entirely sure of the state of their present karma, they always had room for hope and for action. In such contexts, wearing amulets, performing *yadaya* and/or practising meditation provided villagers with a certain sense of agency, control and safety. As Howell noted in his study of the Chewong from Malaysia, 'the embodied knowledge of the prescriptions and proscriptions means that they [the Chewong] experience a profound sense of control' (2012, p. 141). These practices were carried out on a regular basis, a sign of not only the enduring threat and instability of the order but also, as shown by Hamayon (2012) in pre-Soviet Siberia, that fortune was obtained only through an attentive and continual cultivation. This process can thus be compared to the Chinese *yangsheng* (nurturing life) studied by Farquhar and Zhang (2012, p. 269), an ensemble of practices aimed at promoting one's health. These practices were more focused on physical activities, while in Rakhine this aspect was almost absent.

Fear and control

Of course, the sense of control and hence of security has a limit and also largely varies depending on the factors involved. This may explain the special fear many villagers felt for supernatural aggression. Malevolent beings are often invisible and unpredictable, and out of one's control. Contrary to what modernists would argue, this fear, and the belief itself in the supernatural, has not disappeared with education or exposure to modern values. The same has been attested in Thailand by Golomb (1988), who noted that the supernatural remains a potent force in everyday life. The fear of the supernatural over other dangers has also been noted by Desmond and colleagues (2012) in Tanzania. In all these contexts, the concern about bewitchment seems to even increase in the competitive context, which emerged with economic growth.

Another important source of concern, especially for men, is the loss of *hpon*, personal power, which can be engendered by the breaking of gender rules and the contact with polluting objects. Interestingly, pollution is related to inter-gender interaction and hence connected to gender hierarchy. As Douglas (2003 [1966], p. 3) has argued, in many societies, symbolism based on the binary division between purity and impurity plays a central role in identifying danger resulting from pollution. In these societies, pollution often arises from the inappropriate mixing of male and female elements.

Moreover, as Douglas (2003 [1992]) noted, breaching a taboo harms not only the persons who breached it but also those whom it is designed to protect. And for male villagers the danger – and the fear – was higher because they had more to lose; their *hpon* was considered to be greater and while they may be able to control their own actions, they cannot control those of women and they can always become the victim of a woman's actions. The idea of pollution was especially strong in certain rules, notably in those claiming that a woman has to avoid being in a higher place than men, where her vagina will be in a higher position than the level of the man's head; men and women's clothes should be washed and hung separately, with women's in a lower position to prevent men from walking under them; finally, men have to avoid washing women's clothes.

It is interesting that the concept of *hpon*, of local and secular origin, has been revisited in a Buddhist light and associated to the karma. The implication of the *hpon* in health and ill health-related practices contributes to the preservation of gender hierarchies and, in the same time, to the Buddhist system of values and cosmology. Thus, as Douglas stated:

> Some pollutions are used as analogies for expressing a general view of the social [and] many ideas about sexual dangers are better interpreted as symbols of the relation between parts of society, as mirroring designs of hierarchy or symmetry which apply in the larger social system. (2003, p. 4)

Maximising the chances of healing

The ways in which villagers responded to ill health and misfortune were often complex given the high number of factors potentially involved and the panoply of practices and specialists available. The plurality of responses to ill health, as exemplified by the case of Aye Aye, stem from what Pottier has called the 'wish to maximize the chances of healing' or 'to solve all the possible causes of the disease' (2007, p. 141). People were driven by the need to cognitively and practically gain control over the situation and to master the uncertainty. In this distinctly pluralist and syncretic process, there was no fear of a fatal outcome resulting from a wrong diagnosis and erroneous treatment, as is the case in Tanzania (Desmond et al., 2012). Indeed, when the health-seeking process was protracted, new diagnoses were added on to previous ones instead of replacing them, with all treatments deemed to contribute to the healing in complementary yet hierarchical ways.

The presence of imperfect, ambivalent and potentially harmful courses of action complicated the choice, leading people to rely on what they deemed trustworthy. Trust is more likely to develop in relation to approaches which are familiar (Luhmann, 1988) or which conform to Buddhist morality – hence the important role Buddhism has in guiding people's actions. However, health-seeking processes were varied as people's understanding of the threats they faced and coping strategies are largely determined by socio-structural factors (Tulloch, 2008, pp. 152–153), as well as an individual's biography, past experiences and the social context (Henwood et al., 2008, p. 424).

Ambivalence towards Western medicine

Among the several resources villagers used to cope with ill health and uncertainty related to it, Western medicine occupied a peculiar position. Villagers seldom used it to give sense to their disease, neither did they use it much as a preventive tool. Instead, they often relied on it for their curing processes. Generally, people tended to ignore biomedical concepts and the rationale of biomedical practices, but they appreciated the efficacy of biomedical technologies and products.

The low use of biomedicine for prevention and the irregular or misuse of it for curing can be largely explained by the feelings of fear and mistrust people had towards these practices and the specialists delivering them, and by the shortcomings of the health services. Villagers were afraid of medicines and particularly of vaccinations. The fear stems from the very nature of the product itself – its chemical nature – as well as the effects it is likely to engender – side effects and dependence. It is interesting to note that similar fears are common in the modern Western context, as attested by the studies of Britten (1994, p. 466) and Eborall and Will (2011, p. 659) regarding patients' non-compliance with doctors' prescriptions.

These feelings were aggravated by the mistrust generated by the way these products are delivered. This is particularly clear in the case of vaccination, historically perceived as an instrument of control – a form of biopower in the Foucauldian sense (1988 [1963]) – and expressions of false paternalism on the part of the military government, whose commitment to the health of the wider population was generally extremely limited. As shown by Naono (2009), these sentiments had been especially prevalent around the issue of vaccination since its introduction during the colonial period. The absence of trust in healthcare providers represents a serious obstacle to the adoption of vaccinations and other biomedical preventive practices. This confirms the findings of other researchers working mainly in Western countries, which show that 'trust is a key moderating variable between risk perception and decision making' (Himmelstein, Miron-Shatz, Hanoch, & Gummerumc, 2011, p. 452).

In terms of health-seeking process, the factors hindering the access or at least a proper access to the services, largely relate to the services themselves. Services are not only unequally distributed but are also lacking in terms of quantity and quality of staff, equipment and medicines. In addition, they are expensive. Therefore, many villagers avoided using them, or if they did, they were dissatisfied with the diagnosis or treatment.

This situation of the relative inaccessibility of biomedicine certainly contributes to the survival of other practices. Yet, from my analysis, I would not infer that if people had easy access to better biomedical services the other alternatives would disappear, as Skidmore (2008) has suggested. These practices, have their own value and are better able to provide meaning and, in some cases, solutions to problems. This is particularly true for astrology and indigenous medicine. Astrology was particularly valued as it enabled individuals to 'see' their karma, the most crucial factor in the determining their destiny. As noted by Keyes (1983, p. 5), thanks to astrology, the indefinite nature of karma becomes visible, measurable and hence manageable. Moreover, astrology provides explanations that are meaningful in relating disease to the person's position within the world as well as to his/ her biography and destiny. It also provides concrete strategies to cope with the disease and to predict their efficacy. It is a powerful tool in reducing anxiety, giving hope for recovery and imparting a sense of agency. In the same way, indigenous medicine seems to be more effective than biomedicine in curing some common ailments as well as chronic diseases. Hence in Thandwe, even today, the vast majority of people, rich or poor, educated or not, have, at some point in their lives, consulted diviners, astrologers, exorcists or similar practitioners – as all these inhabitants are embedded in a cosmic concept of disease that transcends social background. This also confirms what Dozon (1987, p. 17) has observed that:

pluralism [...and] is indicative of a general level of acceptance of the biomedical model as well as its limitations in addressing all aspects of health (Dozon, 1987, p. 17, my translation).

Conclusion

I found that the local pluralistic therapeutic system was pervaded by understandings of uncertainty and risk as well as by other related notions such as vulnerability, instability and danger. Yet, the system also provided several instruments to cope and thus enhance hope of health or recovery.

As several factors of an unstable and unpredictable nature are understood as contributing to a person's state of health, people live in an enduring state of uncertainty about their vulnerability. The uncertainty is further increased by the fact that these factors can act singly or in combination and that their actions are largely determined by the person's karma, which is for a certain part out of the person's control given that it is also shaped by past lives. But far from being passive, the participants in my study continually attempted, within their limits, to ensure the more or less temporary stability of these various factors that determine health. Because of the important role attributed to karma and the planets people gave these particular attention. Through divinatory practices, they tried to know these factors and, if needed, to 'fill the glass' (of karma) by improving them.

When falling sick, individuals and their families engaged in more or less complex health-seeking processes intended to identify the factors involved and act on them, as only an encompassing action can lead to a complete recovery. This is particularly important in cases of misfortune, for example, when karma and planetary influence are involved. If these are not addressed, the other recourses will remain ineffective. Once again, this is done through divination.

The process is often particularly complex given the high number of factors potentially involved and the panoply of practices and specialists available. The presence of imperfect, ambivalent and potentially harmful courses of action complicate the choice, leading people to rely on what they deemed trustworthy (Luhmann, 1979, 1988). Trust is more likely to develop in relation to approaches which are familiar or which conform to Buddhist morality – hence the important role played by Buddhism in guiding people's actions.

However, health-seeking processes vary as people's understanding of risks and coping strategies was largely determined by socio-structural factors (Tulloch, 2008, pp. 152–153), as well as an individual's biography, past experiences and the social context (Henwood et al., 2008, p. 424).

Throughout the preventive and curative process alike, people were led by hope, a hope based on a deep faith in the law of karma and in the reliability of cosmic norms, and hence on the possibility that the cultivation of luck will bear fruit. Hope was also related to the plurality of options available: in the health-seeking processes, despite the failure of some approaches, a villager could always hope to find another treatment that will work and provide release from disease. Yet, this same karma also represents the limits of that hope, since karma determines the limits of an individual's space of action. However, because an individual can never be completely sure about the state of his/her karma, there is always room for hope. Hence, paradoxically, hope also stems from uncertainty (Brown & de Graaf, 2013).

Whether in prevention or cure, no matter how many factors a person is able to act upon, he will never be totally and permanently protected from disease and uncertainty, because instability and vulnerability are inherent in actors' location in a multidimensional social system. Among the different components of these pluralist health-seeking practices, biomedicine occupies a distinct position. It is highly integrated in terms of curative practices, used in a very limited manner within preventive practices and non-existent in terms of aetiologies. People do not use biomedicine to make sense of their disease; if they do at all, it is seldom sufficient. Preventive biomedical practices are often rejected, as they do not correspond to the local idea of prevention as a regular and constant work of harmonisation with the cosmos and the cultivation of fortune. Biomedicine's role in the system stemmed mainly from its technical power, especially villagers' appreciation of its curative powers, but shortcomings in healthcare services and the dispensing/selling of medicines acted to limit a wider and arguably safer use of it, and were linked to notably risky self-medication practice. This situation is, to a large extent, perpetuated by the substantial obstacles hindering communication between specialists and laymen and a considerable absence of trust between the two parties (Guillou, 2009; Hour & Selim, 1997).

Acknowledgements

I would like to thank all the participants in my study who gave me their time and knowledge.

I am particularly grateful to the experts who participated in my study, as it is often challenging for a specialist to reveal the knowledge and skills acquired through many years of learning and practising. A special thanks to Patrick Brown, Andy Alaszewski and the anonymous reviewers who helped me in improving this text through their reading and suggestions.

Disclosure statement

No potential conflict of interest was reported by the author.

Funding

This work was supported by the Institut de Recherche sur le Sudest Asiatique (Marseille), the Swiss National Fund and the Asia Research Institute of the National University of Singapore.

References

Alaszewski, A., & Coxon, K. (2008). The everyday experience of living with risk and uncertainty. *Health, Risk & Society, 10*, 413–420. doi:10.1080/13698570802383952

Ames, M. (1964). Buddha and the dancing goblins: A theory of magic and religion. *American Anthropologist, 66*(1), 75–82. doi:10.1525/aa.1964.66.issue-1

Augé, M. (1984). Ordre biologique et ordre social: la maladie comme forme élémentaire de l'évènement. In M. Augé & C. Herzlich (Eds.), *Le sens du mal: Anthropologie, histoire et sociologie de la maladie* (pp. 35–92). Paris: Archives Contemporaines.

Benoist, J. (1996). Introduction: Singularités du pluriel? In *Soigner au pluriel, essais sur le pluralisme médical* (pp. 5–16). Paris: Karthala, Médecines du Monde Series.

Britten, N. (1994). Prevention is better than cure, but ...': Preventive medication as a risk to ordinariness? *British Journal of General Practice, 44*, 465–468.

Brown, P., & de Graaf, S. (2013). Considering a future which may not exist: The construction of time and expectations amidst advanced-stage cancer. *Health, Risk & Society, 15*(6–07), 543–560. doi:10.1080/13698575.2013.830081

Chenet, F. (1985). Karma et astrologie: un aspect méconnu de l'anthropologie indienne. *Diogène, 129*, 103–129.

Coderey, C. (2011). *Les maîtres du 'reste': la quête d'équilibre dans les conceptions et les pratiques thérapeutiques en Arakan* (Birmanie) (Unpublished PhD dissertation). University of Provence, Aix-Marseille I, Marseille.

Da Col, G. (2012). Introduction: Natural philosophies of fortune—Luck, vitality, and uncontrolled relatedness. *Social Analysis, 56*(1), 1–23.

Desmond, N., Prost, A., & Wight, D. (2012). Managing risk through treatment-seeking in rural north-western Tanzania: Categorising health problems as malaria and nzoka. *Health, Risk & Society, 14*(2), 149–170. doi:10.1080/13698575.2012.661042

Douglas, M. (2003 [1992]). *Risk and blame.* London: Routledge.

Douglas, M. (2003 [1966]). *Purity and danger. An analysis of the concepts of pollution and taboo.* London: Routledge.

Dozon, J.-P. (1987). Ce que valoriser la médecine traditionnelle veut dire. *Politique africaine, 28,* 9–20.

Eborall, H. C., & Will, C. M. (2011). Patients' ideas about medicines: A qualitative study in a general practice population. *Health, Risk & Society, 13*(7–8), 653–668. doi:10.1080/13698575.2011.624177

Eisenbruch, M. (1992). The ritual space of patients and traditional healers in Cambodia. *Bulletin De l'École' française d'Extrême-Orient, 79*(2), 283–316. doi:10.3406/befeo.1992.1882

Farquhar, J., & Zhang, Q. (2012). *Ten thousand things: Nurturing life in contemporary Beijing.* New York, NY: Zone Books.

Finch, S., & Win, S. (2013). Myanmar health services emerging from decades of neglect. *Canadian Medical Association Journal, 185*(4), e177–e178.

Foucault, M. (1988 [1963]). *Naissance de la clinique.* Paris: Presses universitaires de France.

Gellner, D. N. (1990). Introduction: What is the anthropology of Buddhism about? *Journal of the Anthropological Society of Oxford, 21*(2), 95–112.

Golomb, L. (1988). The interplay of traditional therapies in South Thailand. *Social Science & Medicine, 27*(8), 761–768. doi:10.1016/0277-9536(88)90228-6

Gombrich, R. (1971). *Precept and practice: Traditional Buddhism in the rural highlands of Ceylon.* Oxford: Clarendon Press.

Guenzi, C. (2004). *Destin et divination: le travail des astrologues de Benares* (PhD dissertation). École de Hautes Études en Sciences Sociales, Paris.

Guillou, A. Y. (2009). *Cambodge, soigner dans les fracas de l'histoire.* Paris: Les Indes savantes.

Hamayon, R. N. (2012). The three duties of good fortune. 'Luck' as a relational process among hunting peoples of the Siberian forest in pre-soviet times. *Social Analysis, 56*(1), 99–116.

Hayashi, Y. (2003). *Practical Buddhism among the Thai-Lao: Religion in the making of a region.* Kyoto: Kyoto University Press.

Henwood, K., Pidgeon, N., Sarre, S., Simmons, P., & Smith, N. (2008). Risk framing and everyday life: Epistemological and methodological reflections from three sociocultural projects. *Health, Risk & Society, 10*(5), 421–438. doi:10.1080/13698570802381451

Himmelstein, M., Miron-Shatz, T., Hanoch, Y., & Gummerumc, M. (2011). Over-the-counter cough and cold medicines for children: A comparison of UK and US parents' parental usage, perception and trust in governmental health organisation. *Health, Risk & Society, 13*(5), 451–468. doi:10.1080/13698575.2011.596189

Hour, B., & Selim, M. (1997). Essai d'anthropologie politique sur le Laos contemporain: Marché, socialisme et génies. *Paris, L'harmattan, 'Recherches asiatiques', 13*(5), 433–449.

Howell, S. L. (2012). Knowledge, morality, and causality in a 'luckless' society: The case of the Chewong in the Malaysian rain forest. *Social Analysis: Journal of Cultural and Social Practice, 56*(1), 133–147.

Keyes, C. F. (1983). Introduction: The study of popular idea of karma. In C. F. Keyes & E. V. Daniel (Eds.), *Karma, an anthropological inquiry* (pp. 1–24). Berkley: University of California Press.

Laderman, C. C., & Van Esterik, P. (Eds.). (1988). Techniques of healing in Southeast Asia. *Social Science & Medicine, 27,* 747–750. doi:10.1016/0277-9536(88)90226-2

Luhmann, N. (1979). *Trust and power.* Chichester: John Wiley & Sons.

Luhmann, N. (1988). Familiarity, confidence, trust: Problems and alternatives. In D. Gambetta (Ed.), *Trust: Making and breaking cooperative relations* (pp. 94–108). Oxford: Basil Blackwell.

Mythen, G., & Walklate, S. (Eds.). (2006). *Beyond the risk society. Critical reflections on risk and human security.* Maidenhead: Open University Press.

Naono, A. (2009). *State of vaccination: The fight against smallpox in colonial Burma.* Hyderabad: Orient Black Swan.

Obeyesekere, G. (1963). The great tradition and the little in the perspective of Sinhalese Buddhism. *The Journal of Asian Studies, 22*(2), 139–154. doi:10.2307/2050008

Pottier, R. (2007). *Yû dî mî hèng: 'être bien, avoir de la force'. Essai sur les pratiques thérapeutiques lao*. Paris: École française d'Extrême-Orient.

Pugh, J. F. (1983). Astrology and fate: The Hindu and Muslim experiences. In C. F. Keyes & E. V. Daniel (Eds.), *Karma, an anthropological inquiry* (pp. 131–146). Berkley: University of California Press.

Rosu, A. (1978). *Les Conceptions psychologiques dans les textes medicaux indiens*. Paris: Collège de France, Institut de Civilisation Indienne.

Skidmore, M. (2008). Contemporary medical pluralism in Burma. In M. Skidmore & T. Wilson (Eds.), *Dictatorship, disorder and decline in Myanmar* (pp. 193–207). Canberra: ANU E Press.

Spiro, M. E. (1971). *Buddhism and society. A great tradition and its Burmese vicissitudes*. London: George Allen & Unwin.

Swearer, D. K. (1995). *The Buddhist world of Southeast Asia*. Chiang Mai: Silkworm Books.

Tulloch, J. (2008). Culture and risk. In J. Zinn (Ed.), *Social theories of risk and uncertainty*. Blackwell: Oxford.

Performing prevention: risk, responsibility, and reorganising the future in Japan during the H1N1 pandemic

Mari J. Armstrong-Hough

One distinguishing feature of modernity is a shift from fate to risk as a central explanatory principle for uncertainty and danger. Framing the future in terms of risk creates the possibility – and, increasingly, responsibility – for prevention. This study analyses qualitative data from semi-structured interviews with 20 physicians and 43 members of the general public in Japan during the H1N1 influenza pandemic of 2009 to examine how risk and responsibility were imagined, managed, and reorganised through preventative behaviours. I examined respondents' discussions of a specific preventative recommendation issued in Japan during the 2009 pandemic: prophylactic gargling. I found that Japanese doctors had mixed, often conflicting, opinions about the efficacy of gargling to prevent infection; most felt its usefulness as a recommendation lay in its capacity to give patients the belief that they could mitigate the risk of infection. Doctors who were openly dubious about the effectiveness of gargling in reducing risk of infection continued to recommend it because they felt that gargling provided patients with peace of mind, reducing their sense of ontological insecurity. In contrast, lay respondents saw gargling as a practical, common-sense measure they could take to mitigate risk, but also citing responsibility to others as motivation for performing preventative practices that they would otherwise eschew.

Introduction

One of the distinguishing features of high modernity is the shift away from notions of fate as a central explanatory principle to notions of risk, making the analysis of the perception and management of risk central to understanding high modernity's 'core elements' (Giddens, 1991, p. 114). In 'risk society', the threat of risk has become ever present and individuals need techniques for maintaining their ontological security – their sense of coherence and continuity in the face of uncertainty. One response to uncertainty when normality is disrupted by a major threat is to place trust in and act upon the recommendations produced by systems of expert knowledge such as medicine and public health. However, much of our current knowledge of how non-experts respond to threats of major health events such as pandemic flu and the 'protective coccoon' of ontological security is derived from studies conducted in European and European-derived societies (see, for example, Lohm, Davis, Flowers, & Stephenson, 2015). In this article, I address this gap using semi-structured interviews collected in Japan during the 2009 H1N1 influenza pandemic to examine how risk and responsibility were imagined, managed, and reorganised through the medicalised framing of risk and recommendations for risk-reducing action.

Risk, danger, and the flu in Japan
Risk, prevention, and reorganising the future

Framing the future in terms of risk creates the possibility, the desire, and, increasingly, the responsibility for prevention. Behaviours intended to 'reorganize the future of suffering' (Frankenberg, 1993) seek to reshape the future by managing, trading, and minimising risk in the present; Giddens calls this the 'colonisation' of the future (Giddens, 1991, p. 111). The ongoing reorganisation of the future is perhaps nowhere more evident than in public health, where the consequences of past behaviours are observed and tallied, the nature of present behaviours assessed, and their future consequences estimated and judged. At the individual level, actualising optimal futures in health requires not only the calculation of risk and reward, but ever-increasing responsibility for knowledge consumption on the part of the non-expert (Clarke, Mamo, Fosket, Fishman, & Shim, 2010, p. 23). It is no longer sufficient to merely comply with medical recommendations; patients are now urged to be 'active' and 'responsible' consumers of medicine and health knowledge (Rose, 2006, p. 4).

The intersection between risk and responsibility, then, is both critical to the lived experience of modernity and a key site for public health, which seeks not only to reduce behaviours that generate risk for individuals but also individual behaviours that generate risk for communities. At the same time, as biomedicine and the biomedical paradigm are increasingly woven into everyday life (Clarke, Shim, Mamo, Fosket, & Fishman, 2003, 2010; Conrad & Schneider, 1992; Shim, 2014), new categories of risk and new responsibilities for self-management constantly emerge. These processes simultaneously medicalise what was previously moral (Conrad & Schneider, 1992) and moralise the medical (Boreo 2010).

Medicalisation, risk, and the burden of moral responsibility interrelate in complex ways. The risk categories that health experts produce contribute to a sense of insecurity, while the preventative behaviours they recommend give the general public tools with which to manage that insecurity. But the management of ontological insecurity is not the only purpose for which these tools may be used: risk behaviours and preventative practices may, respectively, produce or expunge perceived responsibility for future suffering.

Japan provides a particularly interesting context in which to explore risk, responsibility, and the reorganisation of the future through public health efforts. Medical anthropologists of Japan, Japanese as well as non-Japanese, have theorised that the underlying symbolic structure of Japanese health attitudes leads to preoccupation with boundary-making between inside and outside, insider, and outsider (see Lock, 1980, 1995; Namihira, 2005; Ohnuki-Tierney, 1984; Traphagan, 2004; Yoro, 1996). Thus, Japanese risk ontologies and techniques for managing them may differ from those of other cultures. At the same time, Japan is unquestionably a society that has undergone the shift to high – or at least 'second' – modernity (Suzuki, Ito, Ishida, Nihei, & Maruyama, 2010), making its study a prime opportunity to examine modernity and risk outside of familiar European contexts.

In this article, I analyse discussions of influenza prevention in semi-structured interviews with 20 Japanese doctors and 43 Japanese laypeople during the H1N1 influenza pandemic of 2009 to examine how risk and responsibility are imagined, managed, and reorganised through medicalised preventative behaviour. The analysis focuses on respondents' discussions of a core preventative recommendation issued in Japan during the pandemic: regular gargling. In the following sections, I introduce the gargling recommendation issued by Japan's Ministry of Health, Labour and Welfare (MHLW); its reception and interpretation by doctors practising in a largely suburban and rural prefecture; and its reception and practice by non-experts in a sample of individuals without health training during the same period.

H1N1 flu and preventative recommendations in Japan

The 2009 H1N1 flu pandemic affected more than 214 countries and territories and was linked to 18,449 deaths (WHO Global Awareness Report Update 112). The first three cases in Japan were confirmed on 8 May 2009, later than in many other affected countries. The 'new type' (*shingata*) influenza stimulated major media interest in Japan. Media attention began in March 2009 and rapidly increased when the World Health Organization (WHO) issued its first outbreak alert (see WHO Global Alert and Response Updates 20 through 49, 2009). Japan's first official H1N1 recommendations came on 25 April 2009 when the MHLW released an 11-page document outlining what was known about the new strain of flu along with a sample notification poster (MHLW, 2009).

In many ways, the H1N1 pandemic demonstrated just how interconnected human communities are around the globe. The various ways in which these communities responded to the sense of acute health crisis, in turn, spoke to enduring differences in the ways that societies and communities envision and encounter the risk of illness. Most nations issued official prevention recommendations, most of them very similar and all of them rhetorically legitimated by biomedical evidence. Most of these recommendations closely resembled the Centers for Disease Control (CDC) model and the WHO's behavioural goals for transmission reduction (WHO Global Alert and Response, 2009). A number of countries, however, added further prevention recommendations. Japan's MHLW added two recommendations to those of the WHO and CDC: the use of surgical-style masks and regular gargling.

These official preventative recommendations were sent directly to physicians and hospital administrators across Japan and passed on to patients. From late April, the Ministry undertook a large-scale publicity campaign encouraging Japanese to practice *tearai* (hand washing), *ugai* (gargling), and *masku* (wearing protective masks). The recommendations were printed on full-page advertisements in newspapers, posted at the entrances to hospitals and schools, repeated nightly on news programmes, and passed on directly to patients by nurses and primary care physicians. Almost every official MHLW communication recommended that members of the public gargle and wear masks and prefectural and city health offices faithfully reproduced the recommendations in pamphlets and public service advertisements.

I focus my analysis on the social construction of gargling as a medicalised risk management practice. Gargling is not the only Japanese recommendation that differs from international recommendations, nor is it a uniquely Japanese practice. However, it is a practice that generates minor disagreement in Japan, generating illuminating conversation and responses in interviews. In Japan, gargling is a preventative strategy buttressed by biomedical authority that is universally recognised but not universally practised. Further, unlike prophylactic masks (Burgess & Horii, 2012; Horii, 2014; Wada, Oka-Ezoe, & Smith, 2012), reportedly used by 63% of the Japanese public during the H1N1 pandemic (SteelFisher et al., 2012), there has been comparatively little social scientific investigation of preventative gargling.

Although it is no longer widely practised as a preventative measure for the common cold and influenza, gargling has historically been associated with influenza prevention in many countries; it is not a uniquely Japanese or East Asian practice. During the Spanish Flu pandemic of 1919, Americans gargled to ward off the flu (Hobday & Cason, 2009). In the first half of the twentieth century, the influential British medical journal *The Lancet* repeatedly published gargling recommendations for the prevention of influenza.

During the Spanish flu pandemic, Japan's Ministry of Home Affairs (1920) described gargling as an international practice and recommended it as one of the main ways of mitigating the impact of the disaster. During the 1918–1919 pandemic and the smaller but serious flu outbreaks that followed in quick succession, local authorities in Japan recommended the use of masks, basic hygiene, and frequent gargling to prevent the flu (Rice & Palmer, 1993). These were precisely the same measures that many individuals in North America were taking – but in Japan an avalanche of public health campaigns reinforced and legitimated these practices and they were likely more widely practised than in North America. Gargling is no longer a common popular practice in the United States, nor is it regularly recommended by American physicians. In Japan, however, it has strong official and medical support and is widely practised – even by physicians themselves.

Methods

Sources of data

In this article, I draw on semi-structured interview data collected from 63 respondents in western Japan during the spring and summer of 2009. The interviews are drawn from a larger set of 115 long-form interviews focusing on lay epidemiology, preventative behaviours, and (for biomedical professionals) experiences and preferences in clinical practice. The analytic sample used here includes only physicians and members of the general public with no health training. Participants who had training in nursing, *kanpo* (Chinese medicine), nutrition, or other health fields were excluded from the analytic sample. Interviews that took place before novel type influenza was a major news story in Japan were also excluded as they did not address H1N1. The time-range specification for each subsample is discussed in more detail below. These exclusion criteria yielded 20 physician interviews and 43 lay interviews.

Recruitment

I recruited doctors in Okayama Prefecture in western Japan using direct requests and snowballing during 11 months of fieldwork in a suburban hospital, an urban welfare hospital, a major national medical centre, and a small private practice. Most doctors were recruited by direct request after I completed several months of shadowing and participant observation in their clinical practice. I recruited members of the public through two snowball samples: one from a rural community served by the medical institutions in which I did fieldwork (mentioned above) and the other from the prefecture's major city, also served by these institutions mentioned above. A rice-farming family with multi-generational ties to the rest of the community and two local teachers facilitated the rural sample. Local librarians at city library branches helped recruit participants for the urban sample by placing cards out at the circulation desk and providing introductions; participants also recommended further interview candidates at the end of the interview. This approach to sampling is non-random and vulnerable to selection bias. However, the use of personal introductions encouraged busy participants to take time out of their schedules for more in-depth, richer interviews.

Interviews

I designed the long-form, semi-structured interview protocol used here to answer a different set of questions for a project examining perceptions, preventative behaviours, and clinical practices associated with type 2 diabetes in Japan. It was merely a coincidence that H1N1 became a public issue during the course of my fieldwork. Because the interview instrument already included questions about general attitudes towards health and specifically prompted participants to describe perceptions of influenza and its prevention, participants naturally mentioned the expected H1N1 pandemic when it became the topic of nightly newscasts and all-hospital meetings. In this article, I draw on participant responses to the questions about general health preservation and flu prevention.

Interviews were conducted in Japanese, recorded, and transcribed in their entirety. The resulting transcriptions were uploaded to Dedoose 2.0, a mixed-methods data analysis tool. Using Dedoose, categorical or quantitative descriptors were attached to each interview indicating the respondent's profession, sex, age range, health training, and urban or rural status.

Analysis

Qualitative codes were applied to identify discussions of influenza risk and prevention. I also applied sub-codes to discussions of each of the most commonly mentioned preventative practices: handwashing, gargling, mask use, vaccination, and avoidance of public spaces. Quotes from interviews were chosen for their representativeness and interpretive potential after coding and translated into English by the author. When I present block quotes from participants in this article, ellipses indicate that the subject trailed off or otherwise changed course mid-sentence, as is common in spoken communication. Ellipses do not indicate that any part of the quote has been omitted. Due to space constraints, the original Japanese is not presented. However, the original Japanese for each translated quote is available upon request.

Ethics

The research protocol received ethics approval from the Institutional Review Board at Duke University. All names used in this article are pseudonyms.

Limitations of the data

The data I use in this article have some limitations; the data collection procedures were developed for a broader research project, which produced the larger subset from which the interviews discussed here were taken. There are three limitations related to the selection and recruitment of respondents. First, the selection procedure for both samples was non-probabilistic, limiting the generalisability of the findings. Second, the sample frame included only those living or working in a single prefecture in western Japan; it would not be surprising if respondents in larger, more cosmopolitan metropolitan areas had their own, distinct perspectives on preventative gargling. Finally, the interviews took place over a period of months (March 2009 to July 2009 for physicians; April 2009 to July 2009 for other participants) as H1N1 emerged as a major cause for concern. As a result, some interviews included in the sample took place during times of real uncertainty, while others took place before or even after H1N1 seemed most threatening in Japan.

Findings

In the following two sections, I examine participants' discussions of gargling as a preventative measure against influenza in the context of the H1N1 2009 flu pandemic in Japan. In the first section, I explore the disagreement among Japanese health professionals about the material efficacy of preventative gargling and why such uncertainty was not shared with their patients. I examine why doctors recommended gargling in the absence of consensus about its efficacy. In the second section, I explore how and why members of the public consider gargling to be beneficial and how they use gargling to manage ontological insecurity in uncertain times.

Doctors, risk, and recommendations

In interviews, doctors described the usefulness of the gargling recommendation as originating from the intuitive sense it makes to patients eager to decrease risk, not necessarily from the belief that it decreases infection risk in a quantifiable way. When asked about gargling, doctors fell into three groups: those who emphasised the empirical basis for gargling, those who were sceptical of the efficacy of gargling and critical of the official recommendation, and those who saw gargling as a uniquely Japanese practice.

However, doctor's belief in the efficacy of gargling did not seem to affect their willingness to commend it to patients; all the doctors in the study stated that they sometimes or often recommended preventative gargling. Further, most doctors expressed surprise that gargling was not used to prevent flu transmission in the United States, which they viewed as a peer country with similar best practices and prevention recommendations. When I asked Dr Watanabe, a thoracic surgeon, why he gargled, he responded: 'Why? Because it's thought to be good prevention, of course. Do Americans *not* gargle?'. In general, the Japanese doctors seemed surprised and mildly troubled that their American counterparts would not engage in such a simple, common-sense hygiene practice.

The doctors who emphasised the evidence supporting gargling referred to clinical studies to explain their recommendations. For example, Dr Nakano, an internist at a private hospital, said, 'Of course I tell my patients to wash their hands, gargle, and wear a mask [to prevent the flu.] This is based on studies at Tokyo University and others'.

A substantial minority of doctors in my sample referred to empirical evidence, pointing out that the practice of gargling had an evidence base. When told that US-based public health scholars are sceptical about the effect of gargling (see, for example, De Vries, 2005), these doctors described studies of the preventative effects of gargling. Indeed, Japanese researchers have repeatedly found gargling to be effective against the spread of community-acquired infections, including influenza and the common cold (for example, see Kawana, Nagasawa, Endo, Fukuroi, & Takahashi, 2002; Nagatake, Ahmed, & Oishi, 2002; Satomura et al., 2005; Shiraishi & Nakagawa, 2002; Yamada, Takuma, Daimon, & Hara, 2006; Yasuhara & Itoh, 1996).

More cosmopolitan respondents were aware that gargling was not widely recommended outside Japan but did not dismiss the domestic evidence supporting its efficacy. For example, Dr Matsue, a paediatrician who had spent several years in Australia before returning to practise at a prestigious Japanese national medical centre, said that she gargled regularly and recommended it to her patients: "Gargling is probably ... There is a variety of research to support gargling. But I think it's probably [just done in] Japan".

She knew from her experiences on research fellowships overseas and familiarity with American and international guidelines for flu prevention that gargling was not a common preventative measure in Anglophone countries. Nevertheless, she felt that she could commend gargling to her patients knowing that it was supported by legitimate scientific evidence.

Although these doctors referenced scientific evidence to support their recommendations, their main rationale was that the practice amounted to common sense – that it *made sense* to gargle. When asked why he gargled, Dr Suzuki, who recommended gargling as a prophylactic for the flu, colds, and a variety of respiratory infections, responded slowly and deliberately: "To clean [the mouth and throat]. Human throats are *extraordinarily dirty*".

Dr Suzuki went on to provide a detailed description of the myriad ways in which human mouths are dirtier than dog mouths. The idea that American health care providers, who spent their time in such dirty professional contexts, did not gargle was mildly disgusting to him. At the end of our interview, when I had turned off the recorder, he encouraged me to try gargling as soon as I got home from my daily fieldwork in the outpatient clinic.

However, the majority of the doctors I interviewed were openly sceptical of gargling's efficacy for preventing flu transmission. Some cited their experiences on medical fellowships abroad to dismiss gargling as a 'Japanese practice'. Others noted that the studies supporting the recommendation were only conducted in Japan. These physicians continued to recommend gargling to their patients. Dr Fujii, a hospital internist, confidently listed the primary preventative measures he recommended to patients, including gargling, using masks, and handwashing. He explained that gargling was thought to work by cleansing the mouth and throat, but also by helping maintain proper moisture in the vulnerable area in the back of the throat. He did not, however, actually believe the practice to be effective at preventing transmission:

> *Interviewer*: Is it [gargling] effective?
> *Dr Fujii*: No, probably not.
> *Interviewer*: Really?
> *Dr Fujii*: Yeah. I think there is benefit in saying it is… there is a sort of sense of security [patients] get from it.
> *Interviewer*: They can gargle and then feel secure?
> *Dr Fujii*: Yes, yes, yes.

While the practice itself may not prevent the flu, this physician still found it to be a worthwhile recommendation because it gave his patients a sense of security. This sentiment – that while gargling might not be effective way of controlling infection transmission, it was an effective way of managing patients' sense of insecurity – emerged repeatedly. Other providers were still less certain that gargling had any benefits. Dr Kimura, an anaesthesiologist who seemed to enjoy his role as hospital iconoclast, stated, "Do I think that gargling effectively prevents the flu? No, it probably doesn't, does it? But, well, we have to tell patients to gargle. If we didn't they would be rather surprised".

Dr Kimura dismissed the information pamphlets recommending masks and gargling that doctors at the hospital were required to distribute to patients during the H1N1 pandemic: 'Medically, I think they're meaningless'. He compared the recommendation in these pamphlets to road signs advising motorist to beware of falling rocks. He noted that the purpose of such signs (and the pamphlets) was not actually to change individuals' behaviour in a way that would prevent their car from being hit by a rock or protect them from catching the flu. Rather, their purpose was to protect the institutions; they could claim that they had warned motorists and patients about the risks, passing the responsibility for taking preventative action to the motorist or patient.

Other sceptical physicians pointed out that gargling made intuitive sense and so they might as well recommend it to patients. Gargling might 'get even a little of the virus out …' suggested Dr Suga, a female internist, adding, 'To what extent it's actually effective, though, I don't know at all'. But because reducing exposure even a little was unlikely to hurt, she recommended it to her patients. Physicians tended to respond confidently that they would recommend gargling (and masking) to patients, but then pause to append a statement such as, 'But I don't really know how effective it is'.

Finally, a small number of physicians grew philosophical on the subject of gargling. Dr Nagata, a cardiologist who, like many Japanese specialists working in small, private hospitals, also worked in primary care, explained, "[We should gargle to prevent the flu because] the throat is weak. I wonder if maybe this is not medicine, but what we learn from our mothers and teachers. But it is also medicine".

These physicians were interested in the idea that gargling was a cultural practice and discussed why gargling might be a particularly 'Japanese' practice. Dr Nagata wondered out loud if the tendency to believe that the throat was weak was related to Japanese mothers' insistence on keeping children's throats warm in the winter, in contrast to American mothers who emphasise keeping children's heads warm. Another doctor suggested that the dryness of winter air in Japan meant that the soft palate of those living on Honshu, Japan's largest island, had historically been more vulnerable to infection than those living in North America or Europe.

Like their colleagues, the doctors who reflected on the cultural factors shaping the practice felt that gargling made intuitive sense. However, they tended to recognise that what seemed reasonable to them might not seem reasonable to their non-native interviewer and endeavoured to explain why that might be. These doctors understood their own medical practice as happening within a particularly Japanese context – they were interested in the fact that ideas about prevention could be so different in other places, but that information did not change their own recommendations. The doctors in this group were sure that the gargling recommendation was a good one *in Japan* and that it was of benefit to their culturally Japanese patients. Whether or not it technically prevented the spread of respiratory infections and the flu they were not sure – but recommending the practice was certainly beneficial to their patients' state of mind.

Whatever their justification for the gargling recommendation, all doctors exhibited a sense of responsibility to help their patients manage perceived risk during a dangerous time. By telling patients to gargle, they believed they were giving their patients a sense of control over their fate. Even if gargling did not work in a measurable sense, most doctors felt it could only help. Thus, regardless of whether or not they personally believed that gargling was effective against the flu, every doctor interviewed actively passed on the MHLW recommendations.

Further, most of the doctors practised preventative gargling themselves. One of the more philosophical physicians reflected on why he and his colleagues not only recommend gargling to their patients with no strong reason to believe it is effect, but also practise it themselves. Sitting in the hospital library on a cool spring day at the beginning of the H1N1 epidemic, he explained,

> Of course, the pharynges are a route of viral entry. Those who gargle ... I think it's good. It ventilates well, too. In truth, for the most part hand washing and gargling creates a *feeling* that one can prevent [illness] ... So in Japan we tentatively enforce the order to 'Wash your hands and gargle'. It's come to be doctors' orders. But even though I say that ... After being out all day, having contact with people with the flu, then after many hours returning and gargling ... well, then it's probably not very effective.

Creating the 'feeling' that one can prevent illness was important for doctors as well as for patients. As Dr Nagata noted even though gargling after hours of exposure to potential infection probably has little prophylactic effect, it gave him the sense that he had some control over illness.

Risk and practice amongst non-expert Japanese citizens

In this section, I examine how ordinary members of the public responded to the medical advice that they should gargle to reduce their risk of infection by the flu virus. I explore the ways in which gargling was imagined to influence risk, how it was used to manage ontological insecurity, and why respondents did or did not enact the recommendation.

The emergence of H1N1 flu in Japan in 2009 disrupted normal schedules, work routines, and plans for travel. Ayumi, an urban housewife with borderline type 2 diabetes, described how the epidemic led her to change plans laid long before flu season:

> I don't really do anything [to prevent the flu.] But this new one, this novel type [H1N1] influenza – [I avoided] crowds. And travel, too. I had plans to go to Korea in May, but I cancelled them. If I went, I think it probably would have been fine. *But if I went and I got sick and gave it to my family, to my daughters – that would be no good* ... It was tough. I had promised my friend I would go. My friend's daughter is also a doctor ... both our daughters are doctors, so I consulted with each and, *not wanting to be a bother*, decided to give up on it. I cancelled my trip one week before I was supposed to go; it was a shame. But I'll probably get another chance to go, so this time I said, 'Let's just give it up', and gave it up. (Emphasis added by author.)

Although Ayumi initially said she had not done anything to protect herself from H1N1 flu infection, she then described changing her travel plans as the flu pandemic made travel more risky. As a diabetic, H1N1 posed a greater threat to Ayumi than to her younger, healthy daughters and yet she framed her decision to cancel the trip as a way of managing risk for her family rather than for herself.

Later in her interview, Ayumi laughingly described how she went to the shop as soon as she heard about H1N1 from her physician daughter and bought a number of masks. But she never opened the package; the use of masks seemed a bit silly to her. However, she did feel there was benefit in gargling:

> *Interviewer*: What about other things, like gargling?
> *Ayumi*: Oh, yes. I gargle. As soon as I come home, I wash my hands and gargle.
> *Interviewer*: Why?
> *Ayumi*: Because, of course, I don't want to get the flu. Because if I get the flu, I'll be unhappy. That's most of it. If it's preventable and unnecessary, if something works, then I should do it. In that way, with no trouble at all, washing hands and gargling has become a daily habit.

Masks may have seemed silly and bothersome, but Ayumi saw handwashing and gargling as sensible preventative measures. Like the health care providers, gargling made intuitive sense to Ayumi in a way that precluded close examination. It was such a simple thing, such a sensible practice, that asking so many questions about it made her laugh.

In their interviews, members of the public described gargling as an obvious, self-explanatory preventative practice for influenza and other upper respiratory infections that did not require justification. Many respondents had difficulty precisely articulating how gargling worked to prevent the flu because it seemed so self-obvious to them. Takumi, a medical supplies salesman married to a non-Japanese women, expressed frustration at his wife's lack of interest in preventative gargling. His wife was puzzled and amused by the recommendation and questioned how it worked, asking: 'How could that [gargling] keep you from getting sick?'. Takumi was so flabbergasted that he found it difficult to explain it to her – the practice was commonsensical to him. Finally he told her, 'When you come home you have to clean yourself from germs!'.

Like the doctors, most of the participants who did not have health training said that they gargled occasionally in an effort to prevent flu infection; most of the remainder said that they 'ought' to gargle daily though they did not. Mothers of young children were the most likely to say that they gargle daily. Junki, the well-travelled wife of a successful businessman, explained that

> Whenever I return home I make sure to … whatever doctor you ask, they will say that the simplest and most effective prevention is to gargle and wash hands. It makes me feel a bit like a pre-schooler, but I make an effort to gargle and wash my hands.

The participants reported that gargling, together with handwashing, was a doctor-approved preventative measure against H1N1 flu. While simple, the daily ritual of gargling was perceived to provide some protection against a feared virus. They rarely discussed *how* it provides this protection even when prompted by the interviewer. They appeared to accept the recommendation because it came from trusted sources: doctors, public health authorities, and childhood teachers.

The association with childhood was common, as most respondents described learning about handwashing and gargling as basic hygiene measures from teachers during their early schooling. Yukiko, a female graduate student in her 20s who lived in the city, explained that, even before the H1N1 scare, hand hygiene and gargling were a daily practice for her in order to prevent colds:

> It's a grade school, pre-school, middle school – a kind of lifestyle guidance you receive during your education. Something you're taught by your teacher. So it's cold prevention, but

it also developed into a daily habit, and I've always kept it up … Hmm? Why do it? Why indeed. I don't really know, but when one goes outside, one might pick up bacteria, so [hand washing and gargling] prevents that. Not prevents, but … if in the course of today I come across some bad bacteria, and I use the Isodine and gargle … if I do that I won't get sick. I won't get a cold. I have never thought very deeply about it. For me it's really just a personal habit, and so I don't really know.

Like this respondent, most people who reported daily or near-daily gargling cited force of habit and instructions from childhood teachers and present-day doctors. Interviewees often first responded confidently that they practised preventative gargling, but then did not seem entirely satisfied with their own explanations of its effectiveness or the mechanism by which they imagined it to be effective.

In their interviews, participants tended to link handwashing and gargling. MHLW notices, prefectural bulletins, and physician recommendations also connected the two hygiene practices, listing them together in singsong rhyme: *tearai, ugai*. Like handwashing, gargling (especially with products such as Isodine) disinfects body surfaces on which germs may accumulate. The fact that interviewees almost always paired handwashing and gargling in their responses suggests that these were thought of as parallel practices, with parallel preventative mechanisms.

For those who did not normally gargle during flu season, H1N1 sometimes presented an exceptional situation. For example, Yuki and Rie, a tax accountant and his wife, said that during a normal flu season, they did not do much to minimise risk. But H1N1 might sufficiently heighten the stakes to change their behaviour:

Rie: In general, we don't really gargle or wash hands [as flu prevention]. But if there's something particular like coming home from having been on the train, then we do it. When we're just back home from a regular old walk, not really.
Yuki: Everyone is healthy [in this household].
Rie: Swine flu [H1N1] is a scarier illness. So if it shows up closer to here, we would probably do it.

In this conversation, Rie and Yuki noted that the seriousness of H1N1 might change their behaviour. But their reported behaviour under normal conditions is also telling: walking around their own neighbourhood was not sufficiently risky to warrant gargling or handwashing but traveling by train exposed them to greater danger and justified preventative actions such as gargling and handwashing. Greater distance and greater contact with strangers were associated with greater danger and thus greater need for prophylactic action.

Consistent with what has been reported in non-Japanese studies (Lohm et al., 2015), participants did not necessarily engage in preventative practices because they believed them to completely or even significantly reduce their own risk of infection. The performance of prevention was a matter of demonstrating conscientiousness. Many women described their motivation for gargling as a desire to protect children, other family members, or even colleagues from exposure. Like Ayumi, the woman mentioned at the beginning of this section, women brought up a wish not to be a source of infection or even 'be a bother' as a primary reason for preventative action. Young mothers reported that after having children they became more conscientious about their own health. These women framed their efforts to reduce risk of infection in terms of conscientiousness and responsibility to others rather than as efforts to reorganise their own futures.

Discussion

As Giddens has pointed out, 'preoccupation with risk in modern social life has nothing directly to do with the actual prevalence of life-threatening dangers' (Giddens, 1991, p. 115). Similarly, I argue that preoccupation with prevention has nothing directly to do with the actual effectiveness of the chosen prophylactics. Creating the sense that a common infection is in some part preventable – that the tools for colonising the future are indeed in doctors' hands – becomes as important as the result of the prophylactic intervention. By recommending intuitive (in the Japanese context) practices like gargling, physicians erect boundaries between risk and security, associating hygiene rituals and attention to vulnerable parts of the body with security and carelessness with risk.

Mary Douglas argued that the erection of such boundaries is a creative, ordering act engaged in through one form or another in all human societies (Douglas, 1966). In Douglas' reading, dirt and disorder are symbolically synonymous. 'In chasing dirt', she writes, 'In papering, decorating, tidying, we are not governed by anxiety to escape disease, but are positively re-ordering our environment. There is nothing fearful or unreasoning in our dirt-avoidance: it is a creative moment, an attempt to relate form to function, to make unity of experience' (Douglas, 1966, p. 3). The construction and observation of symbolic boundaries is neither the result of pathology nor panic, but rather a creative expression of order.

Ohnuki-Tierney's work on the underlying symbolic structure of Japanese health behaviours and attitudes also emphasises the centrality of boundary-making (1984). She argued that the underlying structure of health beliefs in Japan is characterised by attention to boundaries between inside and outside, insider and outsider, based on Japanese spatial classifications. The inside is by its nature 'clean' in a spiritual sense, the outside dirty. In this usage, 'outside' (*soto*) does not refer to natural, 'unpeopled' spaces. Rather, it is a social outside peopled with crowds and strangers, those who do not belong to the household (*ie*). These strangers are implicitly impure: the word for crowd in Japanese (*hito-gomi*) can be literally translated as 'people-dirt'.

The spaces that delineate inside from outside require constant policing and care. In the traditional Japanese home, the *genkan* delineates this boundary; it is the space through which one passes to reach the inner spaces of the home, where one removes shoes carrying the dirt and germs of the outside. In the body, the mouth, nose, and throat delineate this boundary.

Boundary-making spaces are fraught with the uncertainty of being neither inside nor outside, neither completely dirty nor completely clean. They are vulnerable spaces, liminal spaces – spaces that carry the risk of contamination and miscegenation. They are, in short, ontologically dangerous places where inside and outside meet and the threat of pollution always hovers. Just as the *genkan* must be the site of symbolic cleansing and shedding as one enters the home, the mouth must be protected from breathing in dirty, germ-ridden air by masks (Ohnuki-Tierney, 1984, pp. 25–26) and purified through gargling.

The interviews I have drawn on in this article show that physicians and health authorities do not merely *produce* risk through the proliferation of risk categories. Health care providers also *manage* the perception of risk for patients, consciously giving patients the tools to maintain a sense of control over their well-being – the tools to 'colonise' the future, in Giddens' terms. Importantly, these tools make use of shared implicit beliefs and explanatory models that ground preventative practice in a more or less internally coherent symbolic structure in order to help lay people cope. The tools Japanese physicians and public health experts use to do this are rooted in different histories and different symbolic structures from those elsewhere, but they serve essentially the same purpose: coping with ontological insecurity.

Social theorists of medicine have argued that the evolution of biomedicine, and particularly the growth of genetic profiles, has obscured the role of social organisation in individual suffering and well-being (Clarke et al., 2003; Frankenberg, 1993; Shim, 2014). Frankenberg (1993, p. 221) argued that

> The socially and culturally situated and self-situating person excluded already from techno-logical medicine is now being abandoned by curative medicine and perhaps also by pre-ventative medicine.

In the present study, I found that doctors anticipated and self-consciously responded to the cultural context of patient lives and anxieties. The Japanese doctors who professed no confidence in gargling but recommended the practice nonetheless, for example, sought to give patients a sense of control over the future within a particular cultural context in which gargling intuitively aligned with key symbolic understandings of liminal space. Importantly, most of the doctors identified the patients' sense of security as the primary purpose for advising patients to gargle and echoed lay individuals' intuitive sense that the throat was a symbolically important space for cleansing and protecting.

The finding that Japanese doctors report passing on preventative recommendations for the express purpose of maintaining patients' ontological security also has implications for our understanding of the relationships between risk manufacture, risk management, and actors in expert knowledge systems. Doctors valued the gargling recommendation primarily because its practice gave their patients a sense of security, not because of its potential for H1N1 flu transmission reduction, its purported *raison d'être*. Whether or not public health officials viewed the gargling recommendation in this way is not clear, as they were outside the scope of my study. However, it was clear that in everyday practices, official risk management strategies and the risk ontologies they imply were used primarily to buttress ontological security. In doing so, risk is assigned paradoxical meaning: passing on risk management recommendations to patients increased their sense of security precisely because it implied that risk was predictable, that pandemic was containable, that pollution could be confined to the margins with the daily rituals of cleansing and reordering.

Members of the general public who I interviewed were largely unaware of the lack of consensus among physicians and perceived the gargling recommendation to be common sense and authoritative. While some respondents explained gargling in terms of a simple causal relationship, when pressed they were aware that none of the preventative measures guaranteed that one would escape infection. Most viewed gargling as a good habit rather than as a truly protective practice. This is in line with investigations of influenza risk management in the general public conducted outside Japan. Lohm et al. (2015) found in their analysis of interviews and focus groups conducted in Australia and Scotland that respondents valued and reported practising prevention strategies 'even when they asserted that they were not especially effective' (Lohm et al., 2015, p. 124).

The disconnect between the performance of preventative behaviours and the 'actual' efficacy of those behaviours has been noted elsewhere. As risk scholars have pointed out, the relationship between relative riskiness and the emergence of risk practices, or between entrenched risk practices and effective prevention, is tenuous at best (Crawford, 2004; Moore & Burgess, 2011). In the context of another Japanese practice, the donning of surgical masks, Burgess and Horii (2012) have suggested that such practices are best thought of as ritual 'safety blankets'. In the interviews analysed here, gargling, like mask use, generated a sense of security independent of its efficacy. The Japanese doctors noted that the primary function of the gargling recommendation was to produce this sense of security, not to effectively prevent transmission – this helped explain why even those with serious reservations about its efficacy continued to recommend it to patients. The non-experts had received instructions to gargle since childhood, and this contributed to its intuitive, comforting appeal later in life.

Lohm et al. (2015) raised the possibility that individuals taking such preventative measures are aware that they are ineffective but engage in them in part to construct 'a sense of agency in the face of an awareness of being, in strict terms, unable to avoid influenza infection' (2015, p. 124). The non-experts I interviewed did seem to gain some sense of control from gargling in the face of pandemic. And yet the individuals most dedicated to regular gargling were mothers, including mothers of grown children, who often framed their efforts to follow the prevention recommendations as being on behalf of others. These women were not trying to reorganise their own futures; they were demonstrating their responsibility as caretakers of others' futures. This suggests a normative or even moral component to risk reduction strategies: prevention is *performed* as part of a central social role. When risk encounters responsibility, preventative rituals still do not ensure escape from future suffering – they do, however, ensure that if future suffering does occur it can be understood as the result of bad fortune, not of bad behaviour. If so, the ascendance of risk as an explanatory principle has not displaced fortune. Rather, the emergence of risk society has occasioned newly meaningful rituals that (re)affirm the boundaries between the polluted and the pure and, in so doing, (re)confirm distinctions between the blameworthy and the blameless.

Conclusion

In Japan, considerable energy is put into the quotidian aspects maintaining health and preventing disease (Ohnuki-Tierney, 1984; Traphagan, 2004). The Japanese MHLW recommendations for H1N1 flu containment and prevention and the ways in which doctors promulgated these recommendations evidence a health culture distinct from the predominant health cultures of other nations. But these differences in content belie parallel efforts to maintain ontological security in the face of disruption. When infection threatened the population, public health authorities and health care providers produced simple, ritualistic prevention recommendations rooted in daily hygiene practices that were more or less common and commonsensical. The benefit of these practices for stabilising risk ontologies is phenomenological; they hold the power to bring creative order to times of distress, disease, and disorientation.

Risk society in any sociocultural context may necessitate the development of techniques for maintaining ontological security in the face of ever-emerging risks. Yet the content of these techniques can vary considerably according to context. Comparative work on the manufacture and symbolic containment of risk in other modernities foregrounds the social and cultural processes that shape risk ontologies precisely because these techniques differ. The analysis of Japanese practices offered here draws attention to the ways in which the practice and performance of prevention are socially and culturally situated – perhaps particularly for those preventative strategies that seem most commonsensical and familiar.

Acknowledgement
I would like to thank the two anonymous reviewers for their thoughtful questions and suggestions.

Disclosure statement
No potential conflict of interest was reported by the author.

Funding
This work was funded by a grant from the Asian/Pacific Studies Institute at Duke University.

References

Boreo, N. (2010). Bypassing blame: Bariatric surgery and the case of biomedical failure. In A. E. Clarke, L. Mamo, J. R. Fosket, J. R. Fishman, & J. K. Shim (Eds.), *Biomedicalization: Technoscience, health, and illness in the U.S.* Durham, NC: Duke University Press.

Burgess, A., & Horii, M. (2012). Risk, ritual and health responsibilisation: Japans 'safety blanket' of surgical face mask-wearing. *Sociology of Health & Illness, 34*(8), 1184–1198. doi:10.1111/shil.2012.34.issue-8

Clarke, A., Mamo, L., Fosket, J. R., Fishman, J. R., & Shim, J. K. (Eds.). (2010). *Biomedicalization: Technoscience, health, and illness in the U. S.* Durham, NC: Duke University Press.

Clarke, A., Shim, J. K., Mamo, L., Fosket, J. R., & Fishman, J. R. (2003). Biomedicalization: Technoscientific transformations of health, illness, and U.S. biomedicine. *American Sociological Review, 68*(2), 161–194. doi:10.2307/1519765

Conrad, P., & Schneider, J. W. (1992). *Deviance and medicalization: From badness to sickness.* Philadelphia, PA: Temple University Press.

Crawford, R. (2004). Risk ritual and the management of control and anxiety in medical culture. *Health, 8*(4), 505–528.

De Vries, L. (2005, October 20). Does gargling prevent colds? CBS News HealthWatch. Retrieved January 12, 2010 from http://www.cbsnews.com/stories/2005/10/20/health/webmd/main958230.shtml

Douglas, M. (1966). *Purity and danger.* London: Routledge.

Frankenberg, R. (1993). Risk: Anthropological and epidemiological narratives of prevention. In S. Lindenbaum & M. Lock (Eds.), *Knowledge, power & practice: The anthropology of medicine and everyday life.* Berkeley, CA: University of California Press.

Giddens, A. (1990). *The consequences of modernity.* Stanford, CA: Stanford University Press.

Giddens, A. (1991). *Modernity and self-identity: Self and society in the late modern age.* Stanford, CA: Stanford University Press.

Hobday, R., & Cason, J. (2009). The open-air treatment of pandemic influenza. *American Journal of Public Health, 99*(S2), S236–42. doi:10.2105/AJPH.2008.134627 2

Horii, M. (2014). Why do the Japanese wear masks?. *Electronic Journal of Contemporary Japanese Studies, 14*(2). Article 8.

Jansen, M. B. (2000). *The making of modern Japan.* Cambridge: The Belknap Press of Harvard University Press.

Kawana, R., Nagasawa, S., Endo, T. T., Fukuroi, Y., & Takahashi, Y. (2002). Strategy of control of nosocomial infections: Application of disinfectants such as povidone-iodine. *Dermatology, 204* (Suppl. 1), 28–31. doi:10.1159/000057721

Kleinman, A. (1980). *Patients and healers in the context of culture.* Berkeley, CA: University of California Press.

Kleinman, A. (1988). *The illness narratives: Suffering, healing & the human condition.* New York, NY: Basic Books.

Lindenbaum, S., & Lock, M. (Eds.). (1993). *Knowledge, power & practice: The anthropology of medicine and everyday life.* Berkeley, CA: University of California Press.

Lock, M. (1980). *East Asian medicine in urban Japan: Varieties of medical experience.* Berkeley, CA: University of California Press.

Lock, M. (1995). *Encounters with aging: Mythologies of menopause in Japan and North America.* Berkeley, CA: University of California Press.

Lohm, D., Davis, M., Flowers, P., & Stephenson, N. (2015). 'Fuzzy' virus: Indeterminate influenza biology, diagnosis and surveillance in the risk ontologies of the general public in time of pandemics. *Health, Risk & Society, 17*(2), 115–131. doi:10.1080/13698575.2015.1031645

Long, S. O. (1987). Health care providers: Technology, policy, and professional dominance. In E. Norbeck & M. Lock (Eds.), *Health, illness, and medical care in Japan.* Honolulu, HI: University of Hawaii Press.

Low, M. (2005). *Building a modern Japan: Science, technology, and medicine in the Meiji era and beyond.* New York, NY: Palgrave Macmillan.

Ministry of Home Affairs Health and Hygiene Divison. 1920. 流行性感冒 [Ryokoseikanbo/ Influenza]. Ministry of Home Affairs report.

Moore, S. E. H., & Burgess, A. (2011). Risk rituals? *Journal of Risk Research, 14*(1), 111–124. doi:10.1080/13669877.2010.505347

Nagatake, T., Ahmed, K., & Oishi, K. (2002). Prevention of respiratory infections by povidone-iodine gargle. *Dermatology, 204*(Suppl. 1), 32–36. doi:10.1159/000057722

Namihira, E. (2005). からだの文化人類学―変貌する日本人の身体観 [Anthropology of the body: The changing Japanese view of the body]. Tokyo: Taishukan [Japanese language.].

Newsweek. (2009, September). *Hand-washing is no defense against swine flu.* Retrieved from http://www.newsweek.com/hand-washing-no-defense-against-swine-flu-79629?piano_t=1

Norbeck, E., & Lock, M. (1987). *Health, illness, and medical care in Japan.* Honolulu, HI: University of Hawaii Press.

Ministry of Health, Labour and Welfare. 2009. http://www.mhlw.go.jp/houdou/2009/04/dl/h0425-1a.pdf

Ohnuki-Tierney, E. (1984). *Illness and culture in contemporary Japan.* Cambridge: Cambridge University Press.

Payer, L. (1988). *Medicine & culture.* New York, NY: Henry Holt & Company.

Rice, G., & Palmer, E. (1993). Pandemic influenza in Japan, 1918-19: Mortality patterns and official responses. *Journal of Japanese Studies, 19*(2), 389. doi:10.2307/132645

Rose, N. (2006). *The politics of life itself: Biomedicine, power, and subjectivity in the twenty-first century.* Princeton, NJ: Princeton University Press.

Satomura, K., Kitamura, T., Kawamura, T., Shimbo, T., Watanabe, M., Kamei, M., ... Tamakoshi, A. (2005). Prevention of upper respiratory tract infections by gargling: A randomized trial. *American Journal of Preventive Medicine, 29*(4), 302–307. doi:10.1016/j. amepre.2005.06.013

Shim, J. (2014). *Heartsick: The politics of risk, inequality, and heart disease.* New York, NY: NYU Press.

Shiraishi, T., & Nakagawa, Y. (2002). Evaluation of the bactericidal activity of povidone-iodine and commercially available gargle preparations. *Dermatology, 204*(Suppl. 1), 37–41. doi:10.1159/000057723

SteelFisher, G. K., Blendon, R. J., Ward, J. R. M., Rapoport, R., Kahn, E. B., & Kohl, K. S. (2012). Public response to the 2009 influenza A H1N1 pandemic: A polling study in five countries. *The Lancet Infectious Diseases, 12*(11), 845–850. doi:10.1016/S1473-3099(12)70206-2

Suzuki, M., Ito, M., Ishida, M., Nihei, N., & Maruyama, M. (2010). Individualizing Japan: Searching for its origin in first modernity. *The British Journal of Sociology, 61*(3), 513–538. doi:10.1111/j.1468-4446.2010.01324.x

Tashiro, M. (2009). Pandemic flu: From the front lines. *Nature, 461*, 3.

Traphagan, J. W. (2004). *Practice of Concern: Ritual, well-being, and aging in rural Japan.* Durham, NC: Carolina Academic Press.

Wada, K., Oka-Ezoe, K., & Smith, D. R. (2012). Wearing face masks in public during the influenza season may reflect other positive hygiene practices in Japan. *BMC Public Health, 12*(1), 1065. doi:10.1186/1471-2458-12-1065

World Health Organization Global Alert and Response. 2009: Behavioural interventions for reducing the transmission and impact of influenza A(H1N1) virus: A framework for communication strategies. Retrieved March 15, 2011 from http://www.who.int/csr/resources/publications/swine flu/framework/en/

World Health Organization Global Alert and Response Update 20. 7 May 2009. All updates Retrieved March 15, 2011, from http://www.who.int/csr/disease/swineflu/updates/en/

World Health Organization Global Alert and Response Update 22. 8 May 2009. Retrieved March 15, 2011, from http://www.who.int/csr/disease/swineflu/updates/en/

World Health Organization Global Alert and Response Update 23. 9 May 2009. Retrieved March 15, 2011, from http://www.who.int/csr/disease/swineflu/updates/en/

World Health Organization Global Alert and Response Update 38. 25 May 2009. Retrieved March 15, 2011, from http://www.who.int/csr/disease/swineflu/updates/en/

World Health Organization Global Alert and Response Update 49. 15 June 2009. Retrieved March 15, 2011, from http://www.who.int/csr/disease/swineflu/updates/en/

Yamada, H., Takuma, N., Daimon, T., & Hara, Y. (2006). Gargling with tea catechin extracts for the prevention of influenza infection in elderly nursing home residents: A prospective clinical study. *The Journal of Alternative and Complementary Medicine*, *12*(7), 669–672. doi:10.1089/acm.2006.12.669

Yasuhara, T., & Itoh, K. (1996). A questionnaire survey to evaluate the efficiency of gargling. *Sangyo Eiseigaku Zasshi*, *38*(5), 217–222 [Japanese language].

Yoro, T. (1996). 「日本人の身体観の歴史」 [History of the Japanese view of the body]. Tokyo: Hozokan. [Japanese language.]

Purity and danger: shamans, diviners and the control of danger in premodern Japan as evidenced by the healing rites of the Aogashima islanders

Jane Alaszewska and Andy Alaszewski

In this article, we draw on data from fieldwork on the Izu islands and from historical sources to examine the role of shamans in identifying and managing danger and the ways in which surviving practices reflect of the symbolism of premodern Japanese rituals. In most of contemporary Japan, misfortunes, such as illness or maritime accidents, are accounted for, predicted and managed and through modern science-based risk systems such as medicine. However, premodern systems have survived in Aogashima, a small isolated island 222 miles southeast of Tokyo, which forms part of the Izu group of islands. In this article, we use data from ethnomusicological fieldwork on the Izu islands (Hachijō and Aogashima) conducted in the period 2003–2005 and 2010 to examine premodern rituals that address misfortune and uncertainty. We found that on Aogashima, islanders group together a range of dangers such as illness, childbirth and maritime safety and use the skills of shamans to identify the source of the danger, cursing demons, and undertake rituals to counter such dangers by exorcising the demons and their curses. It is clear from documentary sources that shamanistic divination was widely practiced in the Izu islands in the nineteenth century. It is also evident that it was being marginalised and driven underground by the actions of central authorities on the mainland. Given this radical break with the past, the premodern systems in Japan have to be reconstructed from historical documents plus evidence from surviving practices such as those on Aogashima. The shamanistic tradition on Aogashima has become disconnected from mainstream Japanese politics and religion, but it retains a local island-based rationale and functions to identify and deal with specific types of dangers.

Introduction

In this article, we examine the contemporary nature of shamanistic divination on Aogashima and the insights it provides into the identification and management of danger and maintenance of purity in premodern Japan. We show the ways in which fieldwork in a marginalised community, combined with analysis of historical sources, can provide insight into the ways in which elites in a premodern society identified and sought to deal with danger and the ways in which the processes of modernisation resulted in the marginalisation of such responses.

Risk and danger in premodern societies: the case of Japan

Risk, boundaries and pollution

Douglas noted: 'The word *risk* has acquired a new prominence [in contemporary societies]' (1990, p. 1). Increasingly, in modern societies, organisations and individuals see the world through the lens of risk (Kemshall, 2014). All societies have to deal with uncertainty, the challenge of predicting and managing the future, dealing with misfortunes and accounting for and allocating responsibility for past errors and harm. In modern societies, risk analysis has become the preferred response to such issues. It is based on the systematic collection of knowledge about past events, for example, through scientific investigation of disease, epidemiology, the use of this knowledge to predict the likelihood of such events in the future and the use of these predictions to take actions to minimise the possibility of harmful or adverse outcomes. This approach to risk analysis was clearly articulated in the Royal Society Study Group report, which defined risk as: 'the probability that a particular adverse event occurs during a stated period of time or results from a particular challenge' (The Royal Society, 1992, p. 2). Risk management based on risk analysis involves the use of knowledge from the past to provide the context for decisions designed to maximise future benefits. Risk analysis is the basis of systems of decision-making based on statistical analysis to calculate the probability of future outcomes.

This approach tends to underplay both the role of social context and the link between management of the future and accounting for the past. As Heyman, Alaszewski, and Brown (2012) argued, it is an approach grounded in natural science and they noted that each of the core components of Royal Society Study Group's definition is socially constructed:

> Each of the four [core components] can be interpretively reframed, so that 'events' are turned into categories; the 'adverse' into negative (counterbalanced by positive) valuing; 'probabilities' into uncertain expectations and 'time periods' into time frames. (2012, p. 108)

Furthermore, the use of risk to manage the future exists alongside the use of risk to allocate responsibility and blame for past misfortunes (Alaszewski & Burgess, 2007, p. 349).

Douglas (1990) argued that the modern concept of risk performs the same function as religious concepts such as sin did in premodern Europe. Both reflect the structuring of social order and the ways in which threats to it are identified and dealt with. She noted the difference in time orientation between sin and risk:

> From our modern, skeptical, secular standpoint we have the illusion that taboos and sins work backwards: first the disaster, then the explanation of its cause in an earlier transgression. By contrast, risk seems to look forward: it is used to assess the dangers ahead. (Douglas, 1990, p. 5)

However, she argued that just as risk works backward to identify the moral failings underpinning a disaster, so sin works forward as: 'The very name of the sin is often a prophecy, a prediction of trouble' (Douglas, 1990, p. 6).

In her work, Douglas explored some of the shared ways in which different societies maintain order and prevent disorder. She argued that social groups use symbolic systems to represent, think about and manage order and one frequently used system of symbols was based on the contrast between purity/cleanness and impurity/dirtiness/uncleanness. As Douglas (2002) noted, cleanness embraces both modern notions of hygiene, disinfection to kill germs and premodern concepts of ritual purity. Since dirt or impurity is matter out of place, the definition of purity and impurity relies on the proper classification of the world, as the impure or dirty is that which has crossed a boundary and is in the wrong place. Douglas highlighted the importance of boundaries, how they are defined and the role they play in maintaining social order. She argued that the boundaries of the social group had particular potency and that:

> The idea of society is a powerful image... This image has form; it has external boundaries, margins, internal structure. Its outlines contain power to reward conformity and repulse attack. There is energy in its margins and unstructured area. (Douglas, 2002, p. 141)

In this article, we explore the 'energy' associated with a marginal area in Japan, Aogashima island, and how the nature and use of this energy has changed from repulsing attacks on the whole of Japan, to becoming a threat in its own right before finally providing protection for a small, marginalised island community.

Japan and its dangers

Premodern Japan

The Japanese state developed during the first Millennium of the Current Era on a group of islands that follow a north to south axis alongside the mainland of East Asia. Japanese mythology and historical texts stress the autochthonous evolution of the Japanese state and Japanese culture. This development culminated in the Nara period (710–794), in which period bureaucratisation of government led to the establishment of a permanent imperial capital in Nara, modelled along the lines of the capital city of Tang in China. During this period, the central court had a sophisticated literary culture. In the Heian period (794–1185), the imperial capital moved to Kyoto and remained the centre of a sophisticated cultured literate imperial court.

Japan had a multiplicity of religions, some imported from China, such as Buddhism and Taoism, as well as indigenous traditions with pantheons of gods whose ill-will and curses caused misfortunes such as epidemics and natural disasters. The different religions had their own practitioners, for example Buddhism had its monks and temples while 'access' to indigenous gods was through Ying-Yang priests in the imperial court as well as shamanistic experts such as *Urabe* who were mainly located on outlying islands such as the Izu islands, travelling to the imperial court to participate in rituals to identify and mitigate dangers, especially curses of the gods that threatened the Emperor. The orderly maintenance of the premodern state depended on protecting the Emperor and, as Okada (2007, p. 1) observed, anxiety over the physical well-being of the Emperor could lead to instability in the maintenance of the state and, for this reason, it was deemed necessary to quickly unearth any curse threatening the Emperor.

In the Heian period, the danger of pestilence and threats to the health of the Emperor, were associated with menacing deities of outlying areas. These deities were collectively referred to as the *kegarawashiki eyami no oni* (plague demons). The measures taken to identify and neutralise the threats from these gods were based on a symbolic map of Japan in which the demons were kept outside Japan's outer borders. Thus in the Procedures of the *Engi* Era, a Japanese book of law and customs completed mainly by 927 of the Current Era, there is a proclamation that preceded the performance the *Tsuina* rite for the Heian court to exorcise the plague demon. This proclamation sought to neutralise the plague demon by keeping it outside Japan's borders:

The *kegarawashiki eyami no oni* [plague demon] is to be kept beyond a thousand *ri* [a figurative distance] outside the boundaries of these four quarters. The four borders are Sado in the north, Mutsu [corresponding to present-day Tōhoku, north-east Japan] to the east, Tosa [present-day Kōchi Prefecture] to the south and Tōtsuchika [the present-day Goto islands] to the west. (*engishiki* Book 16, the book of the *Onmyōryō* (Yin-Yang) Bureau, in: Bock, 1970)

The *Tsuina* embodies the medieval elites' conception of their world. A symbolic map (see Figure 1) of this conceptualisation places the capital at the centre of a protective square, whose four borders were ritually protected.

The borders of this protected area were situated on maritime frontiers located on the cardinal points. Murai Shōsuke described this symbolic map of the emerging nation as:

A series of concentric circles of purity and pollution extending outward from the capital to the 'external regions' (*iiki*) beyond Japan's 'boundaries'. Each successive zone was more polluted than the last, and the 'external regions' were the most polluted of all, being inhabited by 'devils' rather than human beings. (Murai, 1988, p.111; Batten, 2003, p. 37, English translation)

In the premodern symbolic map of Japan, the Izu islands had a key mediating position between the purity of the central court and the unclean dangers beyond the border. The Izu islands were located in provinces accorded the lowest ranking: inferior and distant. The islands occupied an outer, liminal and dangerous space in relation to the Japanese centre. They were the first line of defence against the dangers that threatened Japan, and the ritual experts, *Urabe*, who practiced on these islands had an important role in identifying and neutralising such dangers.

The islands were also a place where those that threatened the central court could be placed; they were places of exile. The first mythical exile to the islands was the Samurai Minamoto no Tametomo. The Southern Izu island mediaeval *Saimon* (proclamation to the gods), *Kimi no Akachi/Tametomo no Honchi*, described how Tametomo hopped along the

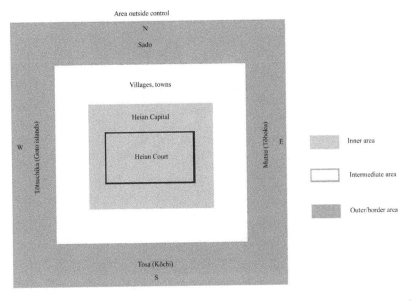

Figure 1. Conceptual map of the Japanese state according to the *Tsuina*. Adapted from Gras (2003, p. 166).

Izu island chain, landing on *Oni ga shima*, devil island, which is another name for Aogashima. Tametomo was credited with the ability to repel the demon of smallpox. He is said to have diminished this demon to the size of a pea and floated it out to sea (see Figure 2). There is in the largest island of the Izu chain, Hachijô, a Tametomo shrine linked to the prevention of smallpox.

While the mediaeval *Urabe* were well documented as they participated in officially sponsored rituals in the capital, there were other ritual experts, some of whom shared the shamanistic skills of the *Urabe* but did not have their full range of skills, for example, male (*Shanin*) and female shamans (*Miko*). *Urabe* had expertise in divination, especially turtle shell divination and boiling water divination, and could gain an audience with the gods by entering trance states and had access to the ritual texts needed in exorcism of curses and demons. Some of the texts were written, but the most powerful ones were secret and had to be memorised. The *Shanin* could also enter a trance state and, though they were junior to *Urabe*, they could become *Urabe* if they could access and memorise

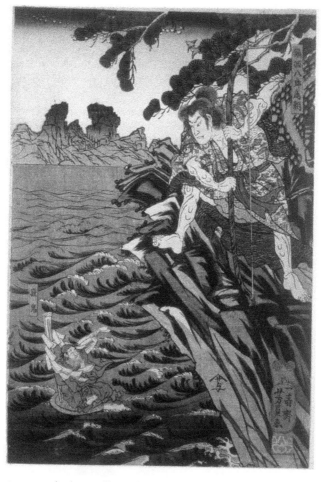

Figure 2.   Tametomo sends the smallpox demon out to sea from the island of Ōshima (Colour woodcut by Yoshikazu Utagawa 1851/1853. Courtesy of the Wellcome Foundation. Wellcome Library reference: 564203i).

the ritual texts. *Miko* could also enter the trance state and cross the barrier between the world of humans and gods (Blacker, 1975/1999, pp. 21–21). *Miko* tended to specialise in a single skill (dance, communication with the dead or healing), though the Izu island *miko* combined all of these skills. There were also *Kannushi* or priests who were usually attached to the shrine of a particular god and undertook rituals relating to that god. They did have the trance powers required to communicate directly with gods and demons.

Modernisation of Japan

From the fifteenth century onwards, the imperialist expansion of European states increasingly impinged upon Japan. Until they were overpowered by gunboat diplomacy in the nineteenth century, the response of the Japanese elite was to protect their borders – repelling the dangerous, unclean outsiders. The external threat was accompanied by internal reform, which can be seen most clearly in the sphere of religion and rituals. In the premodern period, there was religious hybridisation in which Shintō and Buddhist deities were paired and there were joint shrines. The Meiji restoration (1868) initiated a number of religious reforms. These reforms were primarily designed to purify Shintō from foreign influences, especially Buddhism, and to reorganise it to serve a modern state. The reforms created state-sponsored and controlled religious orthodoxy with 80,000 traditional shrines to local gods separated from Buddhist temples and incorporated into a national association of Shintō shrines. The reformers prescribed religious rituals and the ways in which Shintō priests should perform them and proscribed ritual practitioners and practices that did not conform, especially magico-religious practitioners such as the *Urabe* diviners and shamans, who used trances to communicate with the gods and demons. This meant that ritual experts on the Izu islands who practiced outside the formally approved system, such as the *Urabe*, lost their official sponsorship and were persecuted.

The border islands, such as the Izu islands, lost their role as ritual defenders of Japan as the main danger threatening Japan shifted from hostile gods with their curses to European powers with their gunboats. However, the islands did retain one major role, as places to remove and contain members of the elite who were a political danger. These exiles were highly literate and some of them left detailed accounts of island life, including ritual practices. Aogashima's neighbouring island, Hachijō, was a major exile colony during the Edo (1603–1868) and Meiji periods (1868–1912). As such, it was closely scrutinised by central authorities and religious reforms were strictly implemented. During this period, many of the traditional ritual experts left Hachijō. Kondō Tomizō, a samurai's son exiled to Hachijō in 1827, observed in his chronicles of island life, the *Hachijō Jikki*: 'In this year 1885, I write for those who are interested that both families [diviners] have fled and turtle shell divination has died out across the island.' Island ritual texts show that *Urabe* lineages appear on Aogashima and Kojima (a very small island off Hachijō's northwest tip, now uninhabited) at this time, indicating that the *Urabe* fled to these tiny peripheral islands, sheltered by their marginality from the watchful eye of the Meiji authorities.

Traditional ritual experts and practitioners in the Izu islands found their practice threatened in another way. They had traditionally provided services to islanders experiencing misfortune, especially ill-health. Starting in the largest island, Hachijō, this practice was undermined by experts trained in Western medicine. Dutch-trained Japanese doctors founded the first Japanese medical school in Edo (later Tokyo), in 1857. However, doctors began arriving on Hachijō as exiles earlier in the Edo period (1608–1868). This was unusually early for such an outlying community. The *Hachijō Runin meimei den*, a comprehensive record of all those exiled to Hachijō, lists seven doctors exiled to the island in the Edo and Meiji periods (Kasai &

Yoshida, 1975, p. 168). Among these were high-ranking doctors who had served the shogunate. For example, Hosokawa Sōsen, a doctor who worked for the shogunate, was exiled to Hachijō in 1776 at the age of 23 for gambling. He married an islander and lived the rest of his life on the island, dying in 1826 (Kasai & Yoshida, 1975, pp. 167–168). The early arrival of doctors on Hachijō prepared the way for the establishment of a Western-style medical clinic in 1882. Aogashima, in contrast, did not get such facilities until 1962 (Izu shotō, Ogasawara shotō hensan iinkai, 1993, pp. 855–864).

Modern Japan

In the early twentieth century, the Japanese elite had sought to combine features of European imperialism and industrialisation with elements of 'traditional' Japanese culture. This new imperialism resulted in military conquest and expansion beyond the traditional borders of Japan, culminating in an alliance with Nazi Germany and an attempt to replace the major powers dominating Asia: Russia, USA, Britain and France. The catastrophic defeat of Japan in 1945 and the subsequent US influence marked a major shift towards a pacifist, democratic industrial society.

The success of the Japanese economic revival in the post-war era created an affluent consumer society with disposable income. This new-found wealth fuelled a rapid expansion of mass tourism and until the 1970s most of this tourism was internal. In this context, the Izu islands, especially the largest one, Hachijō, became a major tourist destination. It was relatively easily accessed from the major population centre, Tokyo. Scheduled ferry services from Tokyo to Hachijō started in 1910 and were supplemented by scheduled flights in 1955. This enabled the island to develop a sizeable tourist industry. In its 1960s heyday, Hachijō was given the tourist moniker Hachijō Hawai'i. It attracted up to 200,000 visitors a year. In contrast, poor transport links and distance limited tourism on Aogashima. The first regular air service to Aogashima started in 1993, using a small nine-seat helicopter from Hachijō. Aogashima only attracts a few hundred tourists a year (Izu shotō, Ogasawara shotō hensan iinkai, 1993, pp. 308–340).

Other major changes in the twentieth century reinforced the differences between Hachijō (population c. 8000) and Aogashima (population c. 200). We have already noted that the first medical clinic on Hachijō opened in 1882 whereas the islanders on Aogashima had to wait until 1962. Similarly, islanders on Hachijō had an electricity supply in 1927 while Aogashima islanders had to wait until the 1970s. At the time of my fieldwork, Hachijō islanders had been watching mainland television for decades, whereas poor reception on Aogashima meant that islanders' viewing was restricted to broadcasts showing the harbour. Aogashima's Internet and mobile phone reception was poor compared to the coverage on Hachijō.

The different development of the islands in the Izu chain has had a major impact on their social and cultural development. On Hachijō, there is a high degree of integration with mainstream mainland culture. This has led to a reduction in the number of speakers of the island dialect *Hachijō hōgen*, the UNESCO 'definitely endangered language' spoken across the southern part of the Izu islands (Kaneda 2001, 4). There is some evidence of traditional cultural forms such as *taiko* drumming, but this has been dis-embedded from its traditional ritual context, the *Obon* festival of the dead, and has become a form of performance for both islanders and tourists. This has had an impact on the repertoire which has become standardised between *taiko* groups, substantially reduced and separated from the cycle of ritual songs and performance (Alaszewska, 2004, 2009, 2010). The introduction of Western-based medical and psychological

practices has altered the acceptability of traditional ritual practice, such as spirit possession. As Foster has observed elsewhere in Japan (2009, p. 97), such possession came to be
defined in terms of mental illness: possession and related phenomena were increasingly
diagnosed as nervous disorders or diseases of the brain. Those suffering from uncontrolled
possession were not seen as having special shamanistic powers that enabled them to
communicate with gods and demons but were categorised as mentally ill and needing
medical psychiatric care in the newly built psychiatric hospitals. Foster has argued (2009,
p. 96) the psychological and medical concepts introduced during the *bunmei-kaika*,
'Civilisation and Enlightenment' movement of the Meiji period officially altered the
discourse on possession, turning it from an accepted and valued skill into a deviant
practice based on outmoded 'superstitious' practices.

In contrast, Aogashima remains a small, isolated volcanic island (see Figure 3). The
dialect *Hachijō hōgen* is still widely spoken on Aogashima. It does not have a developed
tourist industry and there are no tourist-oriented performances of 'traditional' practices
such as *taiko* drumming. There was also some evidence from the mid-twentieth century
that premodern ritual activity survived on the island. For example, a 1966 documentary
produced by the Japanese national television station NHK, entitled *Ushi to Kanmo to
Kamigami no Shima* (translated: the Island of Cows, Potatoes and Gods), included the
footage of a traditional practitioner, an *Urabe*, performing a demon exorcism ritual.
However given the integration of the island into the modern global community it is not
clear whether premodern belief systems and associated ritual practices have survived into
the twenty-first century. In this article, we examine evidence for such survival and
examine the relationship between these current practices and nineteenth-century and
earlier Japanese belief systems and practices. We examine the ways in which the symbolic
systems that underpinned responses to misfortune and uncertainty remain salient in
twenty-first century Japan.

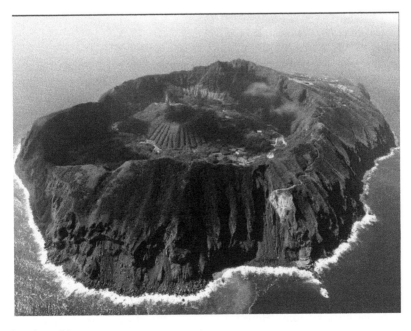

Figure 3.   Aogashima.

Methodology

Design

In this article, we draw on data from several linked ethnomusicology projects. While ethnomusicology research has much in common with ethnographic fieldwork, it has a different focus and different style of fieldwork. Like ethnographic fieldwork, it focuses on systems of belief and practice in other cultures, and fieldwork is based on immersion in the customs and practices of these cultures or as Malinowski described it; 'learning to behave properly' in such settings (1922, p. 6). In the case of the lead author's fieldwork on the Izu islands, this involved speaking fluent Japanese and participating in island life, including learning and playing in *taiko* drumming groups. Similarly, both ethnography and ethnomusicology focus on observing and recording current practices and underpinning beliefs while recognising the potential of historic documents to contribute to an understanding of such practice. Much ethnography has been conducted in communities with few or no written records. Radcliffe-Brown (1958, p. 6) suggested that historic documents could only provide insight into the development of more complex societies over the last three centuries or so. However, Japan with its well-developed tradition of writing and storing documents has a rich store of historical documents that provide information on a far longer time period. In this article we use these documents to reflect on current practices. There are, however, differences between ethnography and ethnomusicology. As Alaszewski (2015) observed, in the early twentieth century, social anthropologists developed ethnographic fieldwork, especially participant observation, to gain insight into the ways in which other cultures resolved universal challenges such as dealing with the uncertainty of the future. In contrast, ethnomusicology focuses on the creation and use of music in different societies. Thus, the focus is on observing and recording the performance of music. As Kunst, in an early text on ethnomusicological methods, noted, a key element of ethnomusicology is the observation and recording of performances:

> Ethnomusicology could never have grown into an independent science if the gramophone had not been invented. Only then was it possible to record the musical expression of foreign races and people objectively... (Kunst, 1974, p. 12)

Non-participant observation is central to ethnomusicology research, and in the studies which we draw on in this article, the technology has moved on from gramophone recording of performances to video recording. This technology enabled us to record and analyse the role of the performer and the audience, the structure and form of the performance and how it related to other performances, both contemporary and historic. As we will show, such data enabled us to decipher the symbolism and magical power of the performance. However, it is important to note that it did not enable us to explore other issues, for example, we were unable to examine how and in what circumstances islanders responded to a misfortune such as illness, using shamanistic performance rather than modern medicine. This is an interesting question but one outside the scope of this article.

Contributing studies

Our starting point was a study of *taiko* drumming on Hachijō. *Taiko* drumming is a well-documented Japanese art form. However, much of the research has focussed on highly commercialised versions such as those deriving from Sado island, which have become embedded in the World Music globalising tradition. There is a commercial element to Hachijō's *taiko*, it is performed for tourists, but there is also strong indigenous tradition of *taiko* historically connected to island occupations such as silk-weaving (Alaszewska, 2009). In her first ethnomusicological study, the lead author participated in *taiko* drumming, learning to play and observing how the groups were formed, developed their repertoire and the contexts in which they performed. She also studied with the last exponent of the island's pre-modernised *taiko* tradition to document a disappearing tradition of song cycles performed in island dialect, which was integrally connected to traditional island occupations (Alaszewska, 2010).

The lead author's work on contemporary *taiko* drumming led on to two related studies, one on historical documents on Hachijō and the other on contemporary ritual practices on the neighbouring island, Aogashima. As we have already noted, Hachijō was an unusual island. Though it was isolated from and marginal to mainland Japan, the central authorities had used it in the Edo period as a place of exile (Alaszewska, 2004). These exiles were mostly educated and literate and wrote diaries and other documents during their exile, often describing the customs and practices of the island. This provided a rich source of material on the island's traditional performing arts and also links to ritual practices in the nineteenth century. For example, Kondō Tomizō, a samurai's son exiled to Hachijō in 1827, wrote about traditional Hachijō ritual practitioners.

The second related study was initially an extension of the ethnomusicology fieldwork to on Aogashima in 2003 to study the island's medieval *Kagura* (plays for the Gods). As the lead author started her fieldwork, the owner of the inn at which she was staying, a female shaman, commenced a 3-day long demon exorcism performance. From her work on documentary sources on Hachijō, the lead author recognised that the exorcism was similar to that which diviners, *Urabe*, had used on Hachijō to identify and counteract the causes of illness. As she further explored the historic sources, it became clear that the Izu islands were a historical base of the *Urabe* and that *Urabe* were present on Aogashima within living memory, disappearing a generation ago. The last known *Urabe*, Hiroe Jihei, died on Aogashima in 1989 aged 90. Working on Aogashima, the lead author was able to identify a number of individuals who were still performing traditional rituals and observe and record some, though not all (she was not given permission to observe and record the traditional rituals associated with death), of their ritual activities.

In the course of her research on Aogashima, the lead author's informants identified a number of ritual sites, mostly in relatively inaccessible locations such as small shrines situated around the island's central volcano's peak. When she visited these, she found the earliest collection of island ritual texts, dating back to 1770. She was also given access to and permission to copy a large collection of ritual texts in the possession of one of the island's *Miko*, Asanuma Kimiko. These texts belong to the family of the last *Urabe*, Hiroe Jihei. Among these texts was a handwritten text of the *Suso Saimon*, dated 1894, written down by the *Urabe* Hiroe Fukujiro (Hiroe Jihei's father). This text was a version of and derived from the mediaeval *Suso Saimon* proclamations to the God of curse (*Suso* is a variation of the term *juso*, the archaic term for curse and the pollution associated with curse). The origins of the *Suso Saimon* lie in the *Suso no harae* purification/exorcism rites of the Heian court (Saitō, 2002, pp. 206–207, 2007, pp. 210–212; Umeno, 2012, p. 349). This *Saimon* text provided an outline of the formula through which Aogashima ritualists counter the *juso* pollution and also a link to mediaeval texts and practices.

Findings

Premodern practitioners: shamans and diviners

Contemporary practice

On Hachijō, we found no evidence that premodern ritual experts were still publically performing, though, as we have already noted, nineteenth-century islanders and exiles to the island did record their activities. During the fieldwork on Aogashima in 2003, not only did the lead author identify a group of traditional ritual practitioners but she was also able to observe the ways in which they used ritual performances to identify and counteract dangers.

At the time of her visits (2003–2005 and 2010), the lead author was able to identify six traditional ritual experts on the island. They were mostly elderly, over 80 (see Table 1), and they may well be the last generation.

The islanders recognised four separate categories of ritual practitioners. At the commencement of the fieldwork, in 2003, the Aogashima *Urabe* had already died out and some of the *Urabe*'s ritual roles have been taken over by the other practitioners. The *Urabe*, *Miko* and *Shanin* all used spirit possession to access the supernatural forces. The term *Kannushi* refers to a priest though the Aogashima *Kannushi* is not affiliated to Shintōism. Once the *Urabe* lineage collapsed, the *Kannushi* largely absorbed the functions of the *Urabe*. The role of the current *Kannushi* on Aogashima is to lead the ritual and recite the ritual texts formerly transmitted by the *Urabe*, accompanying these on the *taiko* drum. However, the *Kannushi* does not perform healing rituals. This is because he is unable to enter the spiritual trance and so cannot carry out the communication and interaction with the Gods which is a central part of the healing ritual.

We found that islanders used these practitioners during 'fateful' moments, when there was a lot at stake and there was a heightened sense of danger. These moments included episodes of serious illness, sea voyages and deaths. The shamans on Aogashima had been initiated and trained by established shamans (Alaszewska, 2009, p. 114; Sugata Masaaki in Aogashima Kyōiku iinkai, 1984, p. 620; Ōta, 1965/1978, p. 78). A key aspect of this initiation was the 'taming' of the god that possessed them. Thus, before their initiation, shamans were possessed, a state called *mikoke* whose symptoms resemble physiological or psychological illness (the latter state referred to as *danshin* ('madness'). In one documented case, *mikoke* manifested itself as loss of sensation in an elbow (Katō 1984, pp. 519–521). The initiation ritual relieved these symptoms so that the god or gods who possessed them became guardian

Table 1. Island traditional ritual experts.

Name	Role	Age in 2010	Additional information
Okuyama Nobuo	*Kannushi*	89	
Okuyama Tomiko	*Miko*	82	*Kannushi*'s wife
Asanuma Kimiko	*Miko*	93	Retired dinner lady, brews local spirits and runs an inn
Hiroe Yachio	*Miko*	95	Died in 2010
Hiroe Kiyoko	*Miko*	85	A tailor, daughter of powerful *Miko* Hiroe Nobue (1902–2001)
Sasaki Hiroshi	*Shanin*	70	Runs an inn

or protecting gods, the *oboshina*. After initiation, the protecting gods resided in the *mibako*, a small wooden box kept in the shaman's house. The shamans were often possessed by Kanayama, a fearsome spirit associated with healing, who is a powerful weapon in the Aogashima ritualist's armoury of healing tools. Kanayama is known throughout Japan as the deity of smithing and metal forging. Associated with fire, the shaman's tool, Kanayama is invested with the ability to change the shape of metal (see Suzuki, n.d.).

On Aogashima, islanders recognised the importance of possession and did not consider it deviant or a mental illness but a sign of the power of the practitioner. Islanders who were not ritualists told the lead author that the unorthodox behaviour which initiated ritualists display was *harusaki*, a demonstration of their power, the Japanese term refers to the transition from winter to spring. (Arai Mayumi, personal communication, 2003).

Historical evidence of shamans and diviners on the Izu islands

Although there is no current evidence of diviners (*Urabe*) on Aogashima, historic texts indicate that diviners and shamans had complementary roles in ritual activity. Since *Urabe* tended to take the lead in ritual activities, the historic texts tend to focus on their role and activities.

The eighteenth- and nineteenth-century islanders and exiles to Hachijō wrote detailed accounts of diviners and their methods of divination, for example, in the *Hachijō Jikki*. The *Hachijō Jikki* (volume 5 Tokyo: Kondō, 1970) begins with a chapter entitled 'Turtle Shell Divination on Hachijō island'. The chapter begins by informing the reader that divination [plastromancy] has disappeared from China but was transmitted to and was still practiced Hachijō. It stated that:

> Plastromancy begins on the seventh day of the New Year. This is called the *tsujiura* of the Seventh. The plastron [shell] is burnt on the fifteenth day. This is called the *ugae*. If there are no auspicious occurrences, then the plastron is burnt during the New Year. Otherwise an auspicious day must be chosen and the plastron burnt. Also mentioned are the preparations of the plastron, its size, the type of wood used to apply heat (cherry tree), and the reading of the divination diagrams. (English translation Hashiguchi, 1994, p. 145)

The *Ennō Kōgo*, written in 1802 by Hachijō islander Takahashi Koichi, contains a section *Hachijōjima kiboku bunji* (literary matters relating to Hachijō plastromancy). The description of turtle shell divination in this section is similar to that in the *Hachijō Jikki*. The *Ennō Kōgo* records that the *Urabe*'s secret texts were transmitted by the house of Akibara; through the *Kannushi* of the island shrines; and the *Urabe* Kaneoku. It observed that the 7-day period during which plastromancy occurred was a period of *mono-imi* (a term for abstaining from contact with pollution). During this period, the diviner underwent ritual purification and had to take precautions against pollution. The diviners had to only eat food prepared on a fire that was separate from that on which food for other people was cooked and had to perform purification rituals to appease the demon gods. The structure of the Hachijō *Urabe*'s plastromancy ritual described in the *Ennō Kōgo* is much the same as the 1691 account of Tsushima plastromancy included in Ban Nobutomo's *Seibokukō* ('Study of Correct Divination'). This indicates that the *Urabe*'s rituals in the three 'border' island centres of plastromancy were based on shared rituals. The *Ennō Kōgo* also provided a chart of the divination symbols which are burnt onto the plastron and an explanation of their meaning.

The *Ennō Kōgo* also provided transcriptions of the two of the Hachijō *Urabe*'s ritual texts. These are the *Yu no hon no uta* (the song of the boiling water divination rite); and the *Shihō Sharui* (Archery of the four corners rite). The *Hachijō Jikki* states that this latter rite was performed at the start of the turtle shell divination rituals held at the island's Mishima Shrine. The *Ennō Kōgo* transcriptions are the only known surviving examples of the Hachijō *Urabe*'s ritual texts. A nearly identical version of the boiling water divination rite is still performed on Aogashima (see Figure 4), indicating that the *Urabe* who left Hachijō in the nineteenth century to escape the surveillance of central authorities transferred some aspects of their ritual practice to Aogashima.

The Edo and Meiji period accounts provided by the exiles and islanders closely match descriptions of the *Urabe* in texts relating to the Heian court (794 to 1185). As we have already noted, these *Urabe* came from the four borders of Japan, and there is evidence from as early as the eighth century that one group came from the Izu islands. For example, an eighth-century box has survived. The *mokkan*, a wooden tablet often used as label on tax goods, indicates that the box originally contained bonito fish (skipjack tuna), which were part of the tax tribute from the *Urabe* on the Izu islands in 746 (Current Era) (Nabunken, n.d.). In the ninth century, a court document recorded that two brothers, *Urabe* from the islands, Hiramaro and Sukune Osada, served at the central court, the former as envoy to China. In the following 1000 years, several documentary sources point towards continuous *Urabe* lineages centred on three of the Izu islands: Oshima, Miyake and Hachijō.

The Heian records show that *Urabe* from the four borders played a key role in the court rituals to maintain the health of the Emperor and counter danger and disorder. They collaborated with other court ritualists, the Yin-Yang Masters, in the rituals to guard the health of the Emperor. The Yin-Yang masters were based in and around the central court,

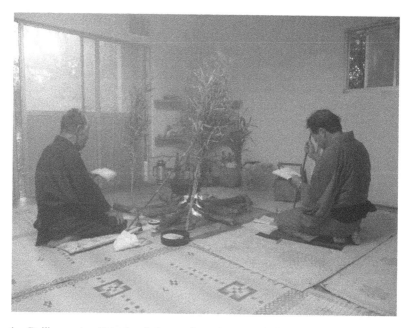

Figure 4. Boiling water divination being performed on Aogashima. All of the ritual participants consented to the recording of this ritual performance. All participants granted permission for the images of the performance to be reproduced for research purposes. The photo was taken by the lead author.

but they did not possess *Urabes'* skills nor their power, which came from living in marginal areas in close proximity to the cursing gods. The Japanese book of law and customs dating from the Heian period, the *Engishiki*, noted the importance of the *Urabe's* divining skills in the following way:

> Those who excel in the divining arts are from three provinces. Five persons from Izu, five from Iki and ten from Tsushima. If they use persons living in the Capital [as diviners] it will not be easy to fill the need from those who excel in arts of divination. (Engishiki book three, page 26, paragraph 5 in Bock, 1970)

Comment

There is evidence that some but not all premodern Japanese ritual practitioners survive and are still practicing on Aogashima. In the next section we will consider the scope of these practitioners' performances now they no longer travel to the mainland to participate in central court rituals.

Premodern magical rituals in contemporary practices

The traditional practitioners on Aogashima focus on the dangers and misfortunes that threaten the islanders. The islanders engage in ritual activities to address three main categories of dangers, those associated with death and the spirit of the dead, those associated with the sea and those associated with illness. The lead author had most opportunity to observe and record rituals associated with illness. We therefore focus on these after briefly discussing those associated with counteracting the dangers emanating from the sea.

Rituals relating to the sea

The fishing communities on Aogashima, in common with other Japanese fishermen, see *Ryūjin*, the dragon deity, as the deity who controls the sea. They pray to *Ryūjin* for an abundant catch and to calm seas, and carry out festivals dedicated to maritime safety and successful fishing, such as the *Shiomatsuri* (tide festival), also called the *Umi no Kuchiake Matsuri* (the 'opening of the sea' festival), marking the beginning and end of the fishing season. These festivals take place in *Konpira* shrine, a place of sacred worship on a headland by the sea. The god *Konpira* is associated with maritime safety throughout Japan. The lead author observed maritime festivals in 2010. Fishermen made a donation to the traditional practitioners who were in attendance at the festivals and also participated in the *Sakuraiwai*, the party which closes the ritual.

Stone markers representing *Ryūgū* adorn places on the island which look out to sea. In addition, the female shaman prays periodically to *Ryūgū*, the palace of the dragon god of the sea. She also recites a traditional proclamation to the tree spirit, the *Kidama Saimon*. As boats were made of wood, the *Kidama Saimon* are connected with boat-making and safety at sea and also have a connection to the prevention of disasters at sea or more generally.

Rituals relating to serious illness

The islanders still consult traditional ritual experts when they are threatened by serious illness. The shamans start the treatment by identifying the source or cause of the illness, which could be a curse from another islander (an *urami*) but, in practice, is usually found to be a curse emanating from outside evil spirits. Such curses can be directed at the victim or can be inherited from ancestors (see Tsuchiya & Horiguchi, 2010, p. 7). Individuals afflicted by such a curse are seen as being in a state of *fujô*, which can be translated as unclean or polluted (*fu*: negative, bad, ugly; *jô*: purify, cleanse, exorcise, unspoiled).

The shamans associate pollution with impurity, dirtiness and defilement. The pollution emanates not only from curses but also from the blood associated with menstruation and childbirth. On Aogashima, menstruating women are considered to be in a polluted state. Women cannot be initiated as *miko* while retaining a menstrual cycle and are prohibited from entering sacred areas when menstruating. Locks of women's hair are placed in boats to ensure safety at sea. However, these locks cannot be taken from women of menstruating age (Sugata Masaaki in Izu shotō, Ogasawara shotō hensan iinkai, 1993, pp. 865–866). Aogashima's women were traditionally excluded from the village while undergoing menstruation, living in *tabigoya* (houses for women in a state of *fujō*) throughout the course of their menstruation, also used as places to give birth. *Tabi* uses the pictograms for 'separate fire'. It refers to the separate fire menstruating women are required to use to prepare food in order to avoid polluting others. The dead are also considered a source of pollution while in the liminal state, which occurs during the period between death and their transcendence to Buddhahood, and there are many rules regarding eating and sleeping arrangements that need to be observed to ensure that the living do not become polluted (Aogashima Kyoikuiinkai 1994, p. 601).

To treat the ill-polluted person, the shaman has to cleanse them by removing and exorcising the evil spirit through the performance of demon exorcism rituals. During these rituals, the shamans call on a powerful array of *kami* (native deities) and Buddhas, using their power to exorcise the evil spirit causing the curse. As the evil spirit is exorcised, the state of *fujô* is lifted, alleviating the symptoms of illness. The entire process is referred to as *chiryô o suru*, or 'treating the illness'.

During her first visit to Aogashima in 2003, the lead author witnessed a demon exorcism ritual performed by the *Miko*. She informed the lead author that the ritual had traditionally been performed over a week by the *Urabe* but she performed the three step ritual over a 3-day period:

Step 1 Preparation of ritual objects to absorb the pollution: Asanuma Kimiko started by making straw boats and figures to carry the curses and their pollution out to sea. The boats were collectively called the *nagashimono* (things floated out). These comprise the *fujô-bune*, (boat of pollution) and the *shichisōkobune*, the seven boats constructed from six small straw boats inside one larger boat (see Figure 5). She also made 49 human-shaped straw dolls, *ura ningyō*. These comprise one large effigy, or 'parent' (*oyakata*) and 48 small effigies. She placed these ritual objects into a cardboard box. She tied straw rope (*shimenawa*) around the box to mark its symbolic status as a ritual space.

Step 2 The Exorcism: Asanuma Kimiko exorcised the demon and its curse by repeatedly reciting over the 3-day period ritual texts relating to purification and exorcism and to the maintenance of safety at sea. To ritually purify the victim, Asanuma Kimiko recited the *Sanju no oharae*. It uses the invocation *Tokami emitame*, the vocalisation used in the *Urabe*'s turtle shell divination rituals. To exorcise the polluting demon, Asanuma Kimiko recited *nokemono* and two *saimon* (proclamations to the deities). The *nokemono* appears to be a unique element of Aogashima ritual. It contains Buddhist components and when reciting it Asanuma Kimiko entered a trance state, performing a repetitive jumping action called *tobu* ('jumping' or 'flying'). This enabled her to communicate with powerful gods who could help her battle the cursing demon. Asanuma Kimiko also recited the *Suso Saimon* and *Kanayama Saimon* (see Figure 6). Both texts invoke the help of powerful gods to battle the curse demon. During the exorcism, Asanuma Kimiko invoked the help of *Ryūjin*, the dragon deity, who can ensure safety at sea and recited the *Kidama Saimon*, which protects against disasters especially a sea.

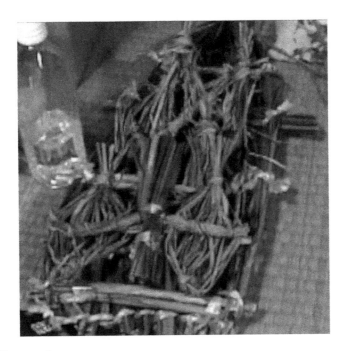

Figure 5.   The straw boats.

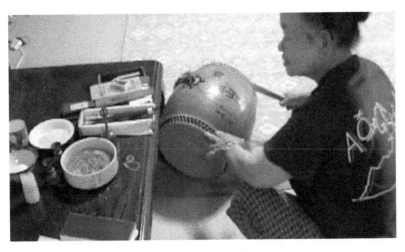

Figure 6.   Asanuma Kimiko performing the *Kanayama Saimon*. All of the ritual participants consented to the recording of this ritual performance. All participants granted permission for the images of the performance to be reproduced for research purposes. The image was taken from a video recording made by the lead author.

Step 3 Casting out the curse: As Asanuma Kimiko exorcised the demon and its curse, they entered the straw figures. At the end of the ritual, Asanuma Kimiko completed the exorcism by placing the straw figures in the straw boats and sending the boat of pollution and the polluting curse out to sea.

The *saimon* which Asanuma Kimiko recited in Step 2 provided a narrative of the struggle which she and her guardian god were having with the cursing demon that was possessing the victim. In the *Kanayama Saimon* she called on Kanayama, the Japanese god of metal work and her main protecting deity.

In the *Kanayama Saimon* which Asanuma Kimiko recited, Suijin, the water god, is a cursing demon and he appears from five directions (the cardinal points and the centre), casting *Juso* curses. Kanayama counters the curses by throwing them into the river, *nagashite harau* (purification through means of casting pollution into the water). The demon king Kijin then appears from the palaces of the five directions riding a *makara* (a kind of sea monster which is also symbolism of the Buddhist *vajra*, a weapon used as a ritual object). Kanayama cuts of Kijin's head. The great evil demon Tenmei then enters from five directions, casting curses. Kanayama repels these. Finally, a list of men and women born according to every sign of the Japanese zodiac appear. Each one casts a curse, which is countered by the all-powerful Kanayama.

On Hachijō, the islanders use modern systems such as medical health care to deal with dangers and misfortunes. On Aogashima, the islanders have a choice. They can use modern systems but they can and do also use systems grounded in premodern beliefs and rituals. They can consult local shamans, who will use their skills in divination and knowledge of traditional rituals to identify and exercise the god that is cursing them.

The historical antecedents of Aogashima rituals

While the *nokemono* appears to be a distinctive feature of the Aogashima ritual, the other texts, the *saimon*, belong to a well-documented tradition of premodern Japanese ritual texts. The *Suso Saimon* are proclamations to the God of curse (*suso* is a variation of *juso*, the archaic term for curse and the pollution associated with curse. *Suso Saimon* and *Juso Saimon* were used interchangeably to refer to the proclamations to the god of curse). The origins of the *Suso Saimon* lie in the *Suso no harae* purification/exorcism rites of the Heian court.

During the fieldwork in Aogashima, the lead author found in Asanuma Kimiko's collection of ritual text a document that provided insight into the development of the ritual symbolism on the island. It was a handwritten text of the *Suso Saimon*, dated 1894 and written down by the *Urabe* Hiroe Fukujiro, thought to be the father of the *Urabe* Hiroe Fukusaburo and hence the grandfather of the last *Urabe*, Hiroe Jihei. This text featured in Asanuma Kimiko's demon exorcism ritual. It provides a narrative of the struggle against the polluting and cursing god or demon. It starts by evoking the God of curses, whose curses are specified through reference to the Japanese zodiac, the *jûnishi*; it then invokes gods for the centre and four points of the compass to fight the God of curse and finishes with the symbolic removal of the curse.

However, the symbolic detail of the *Suso Saimon* is different from that of the *Kanayama Saimon* in current use. Rather than drawing on the pantheon of indigenous deities, it invokes exotic gods from the Buddhist pantheon. It is a form of religious hybridisation that the Meiji religious reforms sought to suppress. These hybrid elements are evident in the setting for the ritual, a Buddhist shrine; the symbolic form of the curse; the representation of the protecting gods; and in the symbolism of the removal of the curse and its pollution.

There is evidence from earlier documentary sources that indicates that current practices and related documents, such as the *saimon*, have a history that dates back to at least the Heian period (794–1185). For example, a document from the Heian court (Saitō, 2004,

p. 163) records a *Suso no harae* exorcism that took place in 972. In this ceremony, the straw figures and boats of the Aogashima ritual were replaced by life-sized objects made from iron, wood and tin. The exorcised curse was placed in and removed by seven carriages with horses, seven life-sized human figures plus the clothes of the person who was the victim of the demon curse.

The symbolism that underpins the current Aogashima rituals was also evident in the major protection ceremonies of the Heian Court, especially the *Karin* riverbank rites and the Festival of the Banquet of the Roads. The *Karin* purification ceremony (see Lomi, 2014) was performed by the Yin-Yang Masters to guard the health of the emperor. In the *Karin* rites, pollution or curses affecting the emperor were transferred to paper effigies. These were placed onto boats and subsequently floated into the water. There are records of several *Karin* rites performed in the Heian period, but the best-known example is the spectacular *Rokuji karinhō* 'Six-syllable Water-facing rite' (Lomi, 2014, p. 276). The Festival of the Banquet of the Roads was connected to the management of pestilence. It was initially held on the 6th and 12th months, but was eventually performed whenever pestilences or epidemics occurred (Philippi, 1959, p. 8). The ceremonies were led by *Urabe* from the outlying areas. In the ritual ceremony, the *Urabe* made offerings of food to the gods where the four main roads from the north, south, east and west entered the capital, to expel evil spirits and repel those seeking to cross the boundary into the city. The Festival of the Banquet of the Roads created a boundary around the city, creating a protective square around the court and separating the pure interior from the dangerous polluting outside.

Thus, the Heian ritual experts, the Yin-Yang Masters of the central court and the diviners from the borders played a key role in protecting the Heian court and its emperor by creating and maintaining the ritual separation of and boundaries between purity and pollution. They maintained these boundaries by performing protective rituals at strategic locations. These rituals cast a square around the court, maintaining a pure centre by casting pollution out into water. An important element in these rituals was *nagashite harau*, purification through water, in which water washed away the pollution. These protective rituals maintained political power by upholding the health of the Emperor and by creating a form of geopolitical hierarchy within the Japanese state. They helped to create and maintain a tertiary political structure consisting of a pure, powerful centre; a middle ground surrounding it; and an outer area adjacent to polluting demons.

Discussion

The survival of premodern rituals for managing danger in Japan

We found that on Aogashima, islanders still can and do access premodern magical rituals to identify and protect themselves from misfortunes such as serious illness. Our analysis of historical sources shows that the origins of these rituals can be traced back to mediaeval Japan, and the rituals practiced in and around the court and capital to maintain purity and protect the Emperor and to define and protect Japan's borders, exorcising and excluding the dangerous, cursing gods that threatened to pollute and harm Japan as embodied in the person of the Emperor. *Urabe* with shamanistic powers from the Izu islands played an important role in these rituals. Through their divination skills, they could identify the source of the danger and play an important role in the exorcism of evil and polluting demons.

The Meiji reforms of religion of the late nineteenth century reconstituted and purified Japanese religion, separating the Shintō gods and shrines from Buddhism and Buddhist temples. The reformers distrusted the shamanistic aspect of *Urabe* and other shamanistic practitioners and therefore outlawed this practice. Despite this ban that affected both Buddhist-influenced texts, such as the *Juso Saimon*, and the rituals performed by shamans, the texts, some of the ritual experts and their performances survived on Aogashima but not on Hachijō. Such survival is uncommon but not unique. In another isolated area of Japan, the mountains of Shikoku Prefecture (a large, mainly rural Island South of Honshū, the main Japanese island), researchers have identified a group of *Izanagi-ryū* ritualists who also use *Suso no Saimon* proclamations to the God of curse in their ritual practices. The rituals of these practitioners tend to draw on the traditions of the Yin-Yang masters of the central Heian court rather than the *Urabe* of the periphery. The discovery of these *Izanagi-ryū* ritualists caused much excitement among scholars of Japanese religion (Komatsu, 1981; Saitō, 2002, 2010; Takagi, 1986; Umeno, 2012), but to date less attention has been paid to the survival of premodern ritual practices on Aogashima.

The changing role of the ritualists who performed these magical rituals, from officially approved protectors of Japan from pollution and danger to practitioners who threatened the unity and purity of Japanese religion reflected the changing nature and definitions of the dangers threatening Japan. In the Heian period, the dangers came from the demons outside the borders, whose curses threatened the well-being of the Emperor who embodied Japan. In this context, the ritualists defined and protected the borders, divining and exercising the polluting demons and their curses. Over time, the dangers changed from hostile demons (invisible to all except shamans) to hostile, highly visible humans. In the thirteenth century, a combination of military force and divine wind (*Kamikaze*) enabled Japan to repel an invasion by the major Eurasian power of the day, the Mongols. In the legends of the Iki islands (one of the 'border' *Urabe* islands), Yurakawa, the local hero who defeated the Mongols, did so by defeating the demons of devil's island (Antoni, 1991, p. 175). However, the expansion of European power from the sixteenth century onwards was more difficult to resist. The Japanese responded to this new type of danger with an emphasis on a new type of purity which was political and religious rather than ritual and magical. Individuals who threatened this purity and who threatened social order were excluded and exiled. The Izu islands had a new role in this new system, they were the marginal places in which dissenters could be placed and managed; they became islands for the exiles. The exiles brought with them the beliefs and practices of modernity, for example, amongst the exiles were some of the earliest Japanese practitioners of Western medicine. This process of social change impacted on the islands in different ways. Most of the exiles were placed on the biggest island, Hachijô. In addition to the practices of modernity, however, the exiles also brought the surveillance of central authority. Both challenged the authority of traditional ritualists on Hachijô. The modernisation of Hachijô continued in the twentieth century, when the island became a major tourist destination and islanders responded to the opportunities of mass tourism by developing elements of their traditional culture, particularly *taiko* drumming, into performances for tourists. Neither the exiles nor the tourists impinged on Aogashima to the same extent and the isolation of the island enabled the islanders to retain their traditional beliefs, practices and ritual practitioners.

Japanese premodern rituals and the nature of purity and danger

Symbolism of purity

The rituals of the Heian specialist and the shamans on Aogashima use the same symbolic logic in which purity is equated with safety but is endangered by the polluting effects of impure, cursing demons. As Douglas (2002) argued in her classic study, *Purity and Danger*, this logic is evident in many premodern and modern systems. Danger arises when polluting impurity threatens to cross the boundary that separates it from the pure. Experts have to counter the danger by re-establishing the boundary and returning the impure to its proper place. In the Heian rituals, the boundaries were spatial, the inner boundary around the pure court and Emperor and the outer boundary keeping the impure in its proper place. In current Aogashima rituals the geographic borders are ritually invoked, but the focus is on re-establishing the integrity of the body of the victim by exorcising the cursing demon that has entered their body. It is possible to see a parallel in Heian symbolism; the body of the Emperor was symbolically represented by the borders of Japan, so preventing polluting demons from crossing the outer borders of Japan also prevented them from entering the body of the Emperor.

Heian symbolism was based on a symbolic map of Japan with the Emperor and his court at the centre and the demons outside the border of Japan. The outermost circle was the boundary between civilised, orderly Japan and the chaotic, unpredictable world beyond, inhabited by dangerous peoples and demons. The innermost circle delineated the court and the Emperor, whose person symbolically represented ordered Japan and any weakness in his body was a threat to the order and well-being of the state. Thus, the focus of ritual practice during the Heian period was the protection of boundaries to protect the person of the Emperor and the well-being of the state. As Douglas has argued, the body is a readily available symbol for society and it is not unusual 'to see the powers and dangers credited to social structures reproduced in small on the human body' (Douglas, 1966, p. 115).

This symbolic system was undermined at the end of the Heian period in 1185, when political and military power was usurped by military leaders, the Shoguns. The Emperor and his court were no longer the only or even major centre of Japan. The Shoguns had their own capital, which, during the Edo period (1603–1868), was Edo (modern Tokyo). The Shoguns were less reliant on magical methods and rituals to protect Japan; their rise to power was related to their ability to militarily defeat and repel outsiders. While the Emperor remained the symbolic head of state, his well-being was no longer central to that of the Japanese state nor was his court the central point and focus of Japan. These political and symbolic changes underlie the marginalisation of the Heian ritual system; from being a national system it became a local system sustained by and serving the needs of a marginalised community.

The demon-exorcising rituals which survive on Aogashima are clearly premodern performances based on a premodern symbolic system in which the inside or body is symbolically represented as an island threatened from the outside by contamination which has to be symbolically returned to the outside, the sea. However, this same symbolism is embedded within some contemporary modern Japanese medical practices. In Japan, public health officials and doctors responded to the danger of the swine flu pandemic (H1N1) of 2009 by advocating gargling with disinfectant (Armstrong-Hough, 2015). Even though many doctors and patients did not believe there was scientific evidence that gargling was effective, they still practised gargling and commended it to others. Thus, gargling can be seen as a uniquely Japanese practice grounded in magic symbolism rather than scientific rationality. Armstrong-Hough (2015) argued that the symbolic power of gargling stemmed from the Japanese belief that the boundaries of the body need to be protected from pollution and that the throat is the major portal, the crucial border-crossing point between the inside and outside of the body that needs the special protection of gargling.

Invisible magical causes of danger and misfortune

In both Heian rituals and Aogashima shamanistic practices, the danger comes from magical sources that cannot be seen by ordinary people and do not operate in the same way and on the same principle as everyday processes. Evans-Pritchard (1937), in his study of the Azande in southern Sudan, found that the Azande differentiated between technical processes such as the quality of the clay and the skill of a potter used in making pots but invoked an invisible magical force, witchcraft, when a batch of pots that had been properly made broke during firing. Heian ritualists and Aogashima shamans invoked cursing demons which they could divine and 'see' in their trance states to identify the causes of misfortune that were beyond the scope of technical knowledge. These experts counteracted invisible spiritual forces by invoking of more powerful forces, their own protecting deities and a range of powerful gods from the centre and four borders.

Danger from within or outside

The Azande looked for the source of the hostile magical forces within their community. Witches were neighbours who were jealous or had a grievance against the victim. When the source of hostility was identified through divination by oracles or the ritual expert, the witch doctor, the witch could then neutralise his or her hostility through a simple magical ritual. In contrast, the Heian Japanese and Aogashima islanders mainly ascribed danger to impersonal enemies outside, cursing demons. They were more like the Lele in the north-east Congo, who Douglas described as blaming misfortune on breaches of ritual purity and on outsiders such as the dead, sorcerers in other villages and those who had left the village. Like the Japanese, the Lele had diviners who could protect the village by identifying and counteracting these sources of danger (Douglas, 1963, pp. 220–258). Like the Heian Japanese, the Lele saw boundaries as playing a key role in maintaining purity, but their main emphasis was on categorisation of their natural environment. For the Heian Japanese, boundaries were a way of dividing and classifying space and place. Their response to danger and misfortune was to use magical methods to identify and protect the borders, to maintain a pure and safe internal space by keeping polluting and dangerous demons and humans outside the borders.

The nature of Japanese division and classification of space changed as the experiences of the dangers changed. As the Japanese elite came under increasing external pressure, especially from the European imperial expansion, so was there increased emphasis on internal purity with the pressure for increased uniformity and conformity. This found its expression in religious reform with the purification of Shintōism and the persecution of practitioners such as *Urabe*, who did not conform to the new orthodoxy, and in politics with the internal exile of members of the elite who did not conform. As Douglas (1970, pp. xxxi–xxxii) noted, changing patterns of blaming reflect changing social conditions. For example, she noted that in early modern Italy the orderly corporate management of Italian city-states was replaced the more arbitrary and corrupt rule of affluent sixteenth-century princes, and the cosmos of those competing for patronage was dominated 'by other dangerous humans competing against them unfairly with demonic powers' (Douglas, 1970, p. xxxii).

Protecting individuals and the community

There appears to be one major difference between the Heian rituals and the current ones in Aogashima. The focus of the Heian rituals, such as the *Karin* purification ceremony and the Festival of the Banquet of the Roads, was on collective welfare whereas the focus of the Aogashima rituals, such as demon exorcising, was on the well-being of the individual. However, this difference may be more apparent than real and may reflect the differential survival of records: the large-scale Heian public events were well documented, whereas the more private and individual activity was not officially recorded. There is evidence that in Heian and later periods, diviners were willing to act on the behalf of individuals. Grapard (1992) observed that in medieval Japan, individuals with sufficient resources paid diviners to protect them when they were undertaking dangerous activities such as travelling overland or by sea:

> As travel was dangerous, safety was ensured by magico-religious practices, the most important of which was divination. Diviners customarily accompanied travellers and were held responsible for their 'projections' on direction, weather, time, and the outcome of their travel. (Grapard, 1992, p. 28)

We have noted that shamans on Aogashima act on behalf of individuals. However, they also participate in collective events, such as the *Shiomatsuri* (tide festival), to enhance the well-being of the community. The situation in Aogashima is similar to that in Zandeland, where ritual experts, witch doctors, focused on the threats to specific individuals. However, Evans-Pritchard also described how before big communal undertakings such as hunts, those involved would ask witch doctors to dance and enter a trance state to 'act as ritual skirmishers to report on and counter the mystical forces of the opposition' (Evans-Pritchard, 1937, p. 258).

Conclusion

Most social scientists accept the view that the technical superiority of Western scientific approaches means that premodern methods of managing danger and misfortune will be replaced by modern systems such as risk management, based on the systematic collection and use of evidence as the basis for rational decisions. Jonathan Miller, a qualified doctor visited Zandeland in 1976 to research and film his BBC documentary, *The Body in Question* (Miller, 1978). He found that 'belief in the existence of witches persists' (Miller, 1978, p. 87) but felt that unlike Western medicine it had a past but no future. In the fieldwork which we draw upon in this article, we found that despite attempts by the central state to eradicate 'deviant' premodern systems, they survived in isolated areas such as Aogashima. Islanders could and did make use of premodern systems of identifying and counteracting danger and misfortune. Ritual experts had the ability to enter trance states in which they could identify polluting demons and could draw on the power of their protecting god and the magical incantation of the *saimon* (proclamations to the gods) to exorcise the demon and its curse and place them in effigies which were sent out to sea in paper boats. In Japan, modernisation of the state in the nineteenth and twentieth centuries was associated with the promotion of modern institutions and responses to misfortune and uncertainty, such as modern medicine. The state has the resources and power to create a new, purified religion and to promote modern, risk-based responses to misfortune and uncertainty. However, there is some evidence of resistance to modernisation, elements of the premodern response to misfortune survive in those communities, such as Aogashima, which lay outside the surveillance of central authorities and in the symbolism that underpins the 'Japanese' ritual of gargling to protect the inner body from pollution.

Disclosure statement

No potential conflict of interest was reported by the authors.

References

Alaszewska, J. (2004). Edo traditions on the 'Islands of Exile': The narrative ballads of the southern Izu Islands. *The World of Music, 46*(2), 99–121.

Alaszewska, J. (2009). *The music of shamans, weavers and exiles: An ethnomusicological study of the performing arts of the Southern Izu islands* (PhD thesis). School of Oriental and African Studies, University of London.

Alaszewska, J. (2010). Two beats to a single drum: Old and new styles of *Hachijō-daiko*. In S. Mills (Ed.), *Analysing East Asian music: Patterns of rhythm and melody* (pp. 1–23). *Musiké*: International Journal of Ethnomusicological Studies, 4, II, 2. Den Haag: Semar.

Alaszewski, A. (2015). Anthropology and risk: Insights into uncertainty, danger and blame from other cultures—A review essay. *Health, Risk & Society, 17*(3/4). doi:10.1080/13698575.2015.1070128

Alaszewski, A., & Burgess, A. (2007). Risk, time and reason. *Health, Risk and Society, 9*(4), 349–358. 2007. doi:10.1080/13698570701612295

Antoni, K. (1991). Momotarō (the Peach Boy) and the spirit of Japan: Concerning the function of a fairy tale in Japanese nationalism of the early Shōwa age. *Asian Folklore Studies, 50*, 155–188.

Aogashima Kyōiku iinkai. (1984). *Aogashima no seikatsu to bunka.* Aogashima: Aogashima mura yakuba.

Armstrong-Hough, M. J. (2015). Performing prevention: Risk, responsibility, and reorganising the future in Japan during the H1N1 Pandemic. *Health, Risk & Society, 17*(3/4).

Batten, B. (2003). *To the ends of Japan: Premodern frontiers, boundaries, and interactions.* Honolulu: University of Hawai'i Press.

Blacker, C. (1975/1999). *The catalpa bow: A study of Shamanistic practices in Japan.* London: Japan Library, Curzon Press.

Bock, F. G. (1970). *Engi-shiki: Procedures of the Engi Era.* Tokyo: Sophia University Press.

Douglas, M. (1970). Introduction: Thirty years after witchcraft, oracles and magic. In M. Douglas (Ed.), *Witchcraft, confessions and accusations* (pp. xiii–xxxviii). ASA Monographs 9. London: Tavistock Publications.

Douglas, M. (1963). *The Lele of Kasai.* Oxford: Oxford University Press.

Douglas, M. (1966). *Purity and danger: Analysis of concepts of pollution and taboo.* London: Routledge and Keegan Paul.

Douglas, M. (1990). Risk as a Forensic resource. *Daedalus, 119*(4), 1–16.

Douglas, M. (2002). *Purity and danger: An analysis of concept of pollution and taboo* (Routledge Classic ed.). London: Routledge.

Evans-Pritchard, E. E. (1937). *Witchcraft, oracles and magic among the Azande.* Oxford: The Clarendon Press.

Foster, M. D. (2009). *Pandemonium and Parade: Japanese monsters of the culture of Yōkai.* Berkeley: University of California Press.

Grapard, A. (1992). The Shinto of Yoshida Kanetomo. *Monumenta Nipponica, 47*(1), 27–58. doi:10.2307/2385357

Gras, A. (2003). Tsuina ni mieru eyami oni ni taisuru juteki sakuyō ni tsuite (sono 2): Eyami oni to ryōiki kettei. Nagoya University. *Issues in Language and Culture, 4*(3), 161–178.

Hashiguchi, N. (1994). The Izu islands: Their role in the historical development of ancient Japan. *Asian Perspectives, 33*(1), 121–149. (H. Mark and Y. Mariko, Trans.).

Heyman, B., Alaszewski, A., & Brown, P. (2012). Health care through the `lens of risk' and the categorisation of health risks – An editorial. *Health, Risk & Society*, *14*(2), 107–115. doi:10.1080/13698575.2012.663073

Izu shotō, Ogasawara shotō hensan iinkai (Ed.). (1993). *Izushotō, Ogasawara shotō minzokushi*. Tokyo: Gyōsei.

Kaneda, A. (2001). *Hachijō Hōgen dōshi no kiso kenkyū*. Tokyo: Kasama Shoin.

Kasai, S., & Yoshida, K. (1975). *Hachijōjima runin meimei den*. Tokyo: Daiichi Shobō.

Katō, I. (1984). Kyōdo geinō. In Aogashima Kyōiku iinkai (Ed.), *Aogashima no seikatsu to bunka* (pp. 487–585). Aogashima: Aogashima mura yakuba.

Kemshall, H. (2014). Conflicting rationalities of risk: Disputing risk in social policy – reflecting on 35 years of researching risk. *Health, Risk & Society*, *16*(5), 398–416. doi:10.1080/13698575.2014.934208

Komatsu, K. (1981). Izanagi-ryū no saimon to Yama no kami no saimon. In G. Shigeru (Ed.), *Shugendō to bijutsu, geinō, bungaku 2. Sangaku shūkyōshi kenkyū sōsho* (Vol. 15, pp. 353–415). Tokyo: Meicho shuppan.

Kondō, T. (1970). *Hachijō Jikki* (Vols. 1–5). Originally written 1827–1887. Tokyo: Ryokuchisha.

Kunst, J. (1974). *Ethnomuscicology* (2nd ed.). The Hague: Martinus Nijhoff.

Lomi, B. (2014). Dharanis, Talismans, and Straw-Dolls: Ritual choreographies and healing strategies of the Rokujikyōhōin Medieval Japan. *Japanese Journal of Religious Studies*, *41*(2), 255–304.

Malinowski, B. (1922). *Argonauts of the Western Pacific*. London: Routledge.

Miller, J. (1978). *The body in question*. London: Jonathan Cape.

Murai, S. (1988). *Ajia no naka no chūsei Nihon*. Tokyo: Azekura shobō.

Nabunken. (n.d.). *mokkan*. Retrieved from http://www.nabunken.go.jp/Open/mokkan/mokkan.html

Okada, S. (2007). *The circular system of rites linking the emperor and the kami-menacing apparitions of the kami in antiquity*. (J. Lefebvre, Trans.). Retrieved from http://kamc.kokugakuin.ac.jp/DM/pdfPreview/Okada_2007.pdf;jsessionid=342F8E159963596E2682AB0C7BD68348.

Ōta, T. (1965/1978). *Ikiteiru genshi shūkyō*. Tokyo: Ningen no kagakusha.

Philippi, D. (1959). *Norito: A new translation of the ancient Japanese ritual prayers*. Tokyo: Institute for Japanese Culture and Classics, Kokugakuin University.

Radcliffe-Brown, K. R. (1958). *Method in social anthropology, selected essays*. Edited by M. N. Srinivas. Chicago, IL: The University of Chicago Press.

Saitō. H. (2002). *Izanagi-ryū saimon to girei*. Kyoto: Hōzōkan.

Saitō. H. (2004). *Abe no Seimei: In'yō no tassha nari*. Tokyo: Mineruba shobō.

Saitō. H. (2007). *Onmyōdō no kamigami*. Kyoto: Bukkyō Daigaku Tsūshin Kyōikubu.

Saitō, H. (2010). Juso kami no saimon to girei: "Jusosai no keifu to Izanagi-ryū "Suso no saimon" o megutte. In D. Lucia & M. Ikuyo (Eds.), *Girei no chikara: chūsei shūkyō no jissen sekai* (pp. 31–65). Kyoto: Hōzōkan.

Suzuki, K. (n.d.). *Kajishin in Encyclopedia of Shinto*. Retrieved from http://eos.kokugakuin.ac.jp/modules/xwords/

Takagi, K. (1986). *Izanagi-ryū gokitō, dai san shū: Ten no kami, onzaki gami, mikogami hen*. Monobe-son: Monobe-son kyōiku iinkai.

The Royal Society. (1992). Risk: Analysis, perception and management. Report of a Royal Society study group. London: The Royal Society.

Tsuchiya, H., & Horiguchi, K. (2010). Hachijo, Aogashima ni okeru Kanayama shinkō: Juso, miko, yamai. *Ningenkagaku kenkyū Bunken daigaku ningenkagakubu* 32, Bunken Daigaku Ningen kagaku-bu.

Umeno, M. (2012). The origins of the Izanagi-ryū ritual techniques: On the basis of the Izanagi Saimon. *Cahiers d'extrême-asie*, *21*, 341–386.

Index

Abelam 29
Africa 2; sub-Saharan 4, 7, 12–18; Tanzania 5, 12–18, 94, 95
Agarwal, R. 43
agriculture: Tanzania 15
air pollution 64, 72, 73, 76
Alaszewski, A. 2, 4, 7, 25, 63–4, 79–80, 93, 119, 126
Alaszewski, J. 5, 124, 127, 128
Albrow, M. 36
Allen, D. R. 14
Ames, M. 80
Amuedo-Dorantes, C. 43
amulets 83, 85, 88, 92, 94
Anderson, A. 63
animals, classification of 30–2
anthropology 4, 13–14, 15, 16, 21–40, 126; beyond ethnographic case studies: accusations, pollution and danger 27–34; classification of animals 30–2; developing the relationship between risk studies and 34–9; development of 22–4; ethnobotany 30–1; ethnography, uncertainty and response to danger 24–7; globalisation 36–9; typologies of societies: magic, religion and science 34–6
anti-Semitism 32
Antoni, K. 136
Anuak 30
Aogoshima *see* premodern Japan, control of danger in
Apostolidis, T. 48
Appadurai, A. 13, 52
Arifianto, A. R. 43
Armstrong-Hough, M. 4, 137–8
Ashforth, A. 15
astrology 84, 88, 89, 90, 94, 96
Atkinson, W. 64
Augé, M. 93
Australia 27, 113
Azande 25–7, 37, 39, 138, 139

Barnett, T. 13
Barrett, C. 69

Bastide, L. 4, 6, 7, 9, 45, 46, 47, 48, 49, 50
Batten, B. 121
Bauböck, R. 47
Beattie, J. 22
Beck, U. 2, 3, 5, 6, 8, 13, 14, 44, 62–3, 64, 65, 66, 67, 70, 71, 72, 73, 75, 76
Becker, H. S. 48
Benoist, J. 93
Bertaux, D. 48
Bertrand, R. 50, 55
Bible: Deuteronomy 31; Leviticus 31, 32; Romans 8
Bigo, D. 43
biomedicine 8, 16–17, 18, 102, 103, 113; Myanmar 80, 82, 85, 89, 92, 93, 95–7, 98
Blacker, C. 123
Blaikie, P. 63
Bloor, M. 13
Bock, F. G. 121, 131
Boholm, A. 13
Boreo, N. 102
Bostrom, M. 16
Boudicca 22
boundaries 4–5, 32, 67, 102, 112, 114, 119–20, 138; premodern Japan 119–21, 135, 136, 137–8
Bourdieu, P. 17, 33–4
Boyne, R. 17
Brazil 27
breast-feeding 8
bricolaging or syncretic approaches 3, 9
Brinkman, J. 70, 71
Britten, N. 96
Brown, P. 8, 35, 97
Brubaker, R. 2
Buddhism 6, 8, 80, 82, 83, 85, 86, 87, 88, 89, 90, 92–3, 95, 97; Japan 120, 123, 132, 134, 136
Bujra, J. 13
Bulmer, R. 30–1
Burgess, A. 103, 114

Caesar, J. 22
Caljouw, M. 71

cancer 8
Candea, M. 48
Caplan, P. 16, 65
Castells, M. 45
Chenet, F. 94
children 7; vaccinations 89, 96
China 34–5; *yangsheng* (nurturing life) 94
Clarke, A. 102, 113
class 62, 63, 64, 72, 73, 75–6; Myanmar 86
climate change/global warming 63, 64, 65, 72–3, 76
Coates, T. J. 13
Coderey, C. 3, 6, 7, 8, 9, 80, 88
colonialism 4, 13, 14, 36, 76, 80, 96
Comaroff, J. 15
Conrad, P. 102
Crawford, R. 113
cultural attitudes towards risk 65
cultural contingency 12–18
cultural hybridisation 39
cultural identity, life style and risk: Sámi women 37–8
cultural practice of gargling 4–5, 108, 113
Curran, D. 64
Cybriwsky, R. 70

Da Gol, G. 94
De Vries, L. 106
Dengue fever 67, 69, 76
Desmond, N. 2, 5, 6, 7, 16, 17, 94, 95
Dickens, P. 65, 76
dietary rules 88, 90
Dilger, H. 13
divination 5, 17, 34, 39; Japan 122, 123, 128–31, 132, 134, 135, 136, 138, 139; Rakhine (Myanmar) 82, 88–9, 90–1, 92, 96, 97
Dodier, N. 48
Douglas, M. 2, 4, 5, 13, 14, 16–17, 26, 28, 29–30, 31–3, 34, 39, 64, 65, 66–7, 73, 74, 76, 80, 94–5, 112, 119–20, 137, 138–9
Dozon, J.-P. 96–7
Drabble, J. H. 45
Durkheim, E. 27

Eborall, H. C. 96
ecological prevention paradox 7–8
economics 43
Einarsdottir, J. 14
Eisenbruch, M. 80, 93
England 32, 35, 63
Enlightenment 3
environmental pollution 65
Evans-Pritchard, E. E. 7, 14, 25–7, 29, 39, 138, 139
Ewald, F. 58
exchange 28, 29, 33–4; and gift 27
exorcism 5, 91, 92–3, 96, 122, 125, 127, 132–5, 136, 137, 139

Faircloth, C. 8
Faist, T. 43
Falzon, M.-A. 47, 48
Farmer, P. 13
Farquhar, J. 94
Fassin, D. 54
Favret-Saada, J. 7, 57
Finch, S. 80
Fischoff, B. 13
flood risk *see* Indonesia and application of risk society thesis: flood risk and poverty in Jakarta
flu pandemic (H1N1) in Japan 4–5, 101–14, 137–8; discussion 112–14; findings 106–11; methods 104–6; preventative recommendations 103–4; risk, prevention and reorganising the future 102–3
Ford, M. 43, 47
Forge, A. 29
Foster, M. D. 125
Foucault, M. 1, 2, 13, 46, 96
framing 4, 102, 111; cultural contingency 12–18; Indonesian labour migrants 43, 44, 51, 52, 56
France 1, 2, 7, 27, 57, 124
Frankenberg, R. 102, 113
Frazer, S. 22–3
French Guyana 1, 67
functionalism 14
Furedi, F. 63

Gale, N. 8
Garcés-Mascareñas, B. 43, 47
Garfinkel, H. 48, 49
gargling 140; flu pandemic (H1N1) in Japan *see separate entry*
Geertz, C. 14
Geissler, W. 14
Gellner, D. N. 80
gender hierarchies 65, 94–5
gender roles 67
Germany 2, 3, 65, 67, 76, 124
Geshiere, P. 15
Giddens, A. 2, 3, 6, 8, 13, 15, 16, 44, 65, 101, 102, 112
gift and exchange *see* exchange
Gjernes, T. 37–8
Glaser, B. G. 48
global warming/climate change 63, 64, 65, 72–3, 76
globalisation 6, 14, 18, 34, 45; definition 36; magic, religion and 36–9; risk society and 62, 63, 65–6; World Music 127
Goffman, E. 48, 49, 51
Goldthorpe, J. H. 64
Golomb, L. 80, 94
Gombrich, R. 94
governmentality 1, 2, 43

144

Grapard, A. 139
Greece, ancient 22, 34–5
Green, J. 18, 26
Guenzi, C. 84
Guillou, A. Y. 98

H1N1 influenza pandemic in Japan 4–5,
    101–14, 137–8, 140
Habermas, J. 2, 7
Haddon, A. C. 23
Hamayon, R. N. 94
hand washing 103, 106, 107, 109, 110–11
Hart, G. 16
Hart, K. 22, 24
Hashiguchi, N. 129
Hayashi, Y. 80
Henwood, K. 13, 16, 80, 95, 97
Herle, A. 23, 36
Heyman, B. 3, 8, 119
Hima people 67
Himmelstein, M. 96
Hiroe Jihei 127, 134
HIV/AIDS 13, 14, 15, 16, 18
Hobday, R. 104
Hobsbawn, E. 15
Horii, M. 103
Horlick-Jones, T. 3, 9
hospitals: tuberculosis 7, 38–9
Hour, B. 98
Howell, S. L. 94
Hughes, E. C. 49
Huysmans, J. 43

immunisation 89, 96
indigenous medicine 80, 82, 92, 93, 96
Indonesia and application of risk society thesis:
    flood risk and poverty in Jakarta 5, 62–76;
    applicability of risk society theory outside
    late-modern society 62–7; discussion 75–6;
    findings 70–5; methodology 68–70
Indonesian labour migrants: faith and
    uncertainty 6, 42–58; findings 50–6;
    methodology 47–9; risk and migration 43–7;
    risk and mixed rationalities 56–8
influenza pandemic (H1N1) in Japan 4–5,
    101–14, 137–8, 140; discussion 112–14;
    findings 106–11; methods 104–6; preventative
    recommendations 103–4, 114; risk, prevention
    and reorganising the future 102–3
insiders 32, 35, 64, 102, 112
intestinal worms (mchango) 17
intra-disciplinarity of risk 14
Irwin, A. 66
Italy 138–9

Japan 34–5, 36; control of danger in premodern
    5, 118–40; influenza pandemic (H1N1) 4–5,
    101–14, 137–8

Jerolmack, C. 48
Jews 32, 35, 67

Kadri, T. 71
Kaneda, A. 124
Karm people 30–1
karma 6, 83–6, 87, 88, 89–90, 92, 94, 95, 96, 97
Karp, I. 13
Kasai, S. 123–4
Katō, I. 128
Kaur, A. 43
Kawana, R. 106
Kemshall, H. 119
Keyes, C. F. 96
Keynes, J. M. 25
Kierkegaard, S. 8
Killias, O. 43
Komatsu, K. 136
Kondō, T. 129
Krause, K. 8
Kunst, J. 126

Laderman, C. C. 93
language: linguistic relevance of risk in
    sub-Saharan Africa 12, 14–16, 18
Le Breton, D. 44
Leach, E. R. 28–9
Lefebvre, H. 47
Lele 29, 31, 33, 39, 138
Lévi-Strauss, C. 27–9, 33, 36
Levitt, P. 47
Lewis, I. 7
Lienhardt, G. 30
Lindquist, J. A. 43, 47
Lock, M. 102
Lockhart, C. 13
Lohm, D. 101, 111, 113, 114
Lomi, B. 135
Low, L. 45
Luhmann, N. 63, 95, 97
Lupton, D. 13, 14, 16, 33
Lyng, S. 6

McCarthy, P. 70
Macfarlane, A. 15, 34, 35–6
magic 3, 4, 7–8, 9, 28, 29, 32, 40; Azande 27;
    Frazer 22–3; globalisation, religion and 36–9;
    Indonesian labour migrants 50, 57; Japan
    123, 126, 131–5, 136, 137, 138, 139;
    Trobriand Islanders: technology and 4, 24–5;
    typologies of societies: religion, science and
    34–6
malaria 17
Malaysia 94; Indonesian labour migrants 42–58
Malinowski, B. 4, 9, 23–5, 27, 33, 36, 37, 39,
    126
Marcus, G. E. 47
Marfai, M. A. 70

INDEX

Martinique 1, 67
masks 38–9; flu pandemic (H1N1) in Japan
    103–4, 105, 106, 107, 108, 109–10, 112, 114
Massenzio, M. 28, 36
Massey, D. B. 47
Massey, D. S. 43
Mauss, M. 27–8, 33
Mazzucato, V. 43
menstruation 83, 84, 132
mental illness 125, 129
method and risk perception 12, 14, 16–17, 18
Michael, C. 68
Mieulet, E. 1, 67, 76
migration: Indonesian labour migrants 6,
    42–58; destiny and sense-making 54–6;
    findings 50–6; methodology 47–9; migration
    and religious response to danger and
    uncertainty 50–2; migration routes:
    manufactured uncertainties and lived
    experiences of vulnerability 45–7; risk,
    agency, responsibility 52–4; risk and mixed
    rationalities 56–8; risk and rationality 43–5;
    ritual meals 50
Miller, J. 37, 139
Moore, S. E. H. 113
mosquito control 67
Murai, S. 121
music 126–7, 128, 136
Myanmar: coping with health-related
    uncertainties and risks in Rakhine 6, 8,
    79–98; biomedicine 80, 82, 85, 89, 92, 93,
    95–7, 98; Buddhism 6, 80, 82, 83, 85, 86, 87,
    88, 89, 90, 92–3, 95, 97; dealing with risk of
    disease: preventive practices 86–90; dietary
    rules 88, 90; discussion 93–7; divination 82,
    88–9, 90–1, 92, 96, 97; exorcists 91, 92–3,
    96; findings 83–93; health, risk and
    therapeutic pluralism 79–81; hope 86, 92,
    93–4, 96, 97; karma 6, 83–6, 87, 88, 89–90,
    92, 94, 95, 96, 97; local aetiological system
    83–5; local aetiologies, uncertainty,
    instability and unpredictability of 85–6;
    methodology 81–3; personal power (hpon)
    84, 94–5; pharmaceuticals 93; planetary
    influence (gyo) 84, 85, 88, 89, 90, 92, 96, 97;
    respect of supernatural and preventive action
    87; respecting social order and conventions
    87; responding to disease: uncertainty in
    caring process 90–3; spirits 84, 87, 90–1;
    trust 92, 95, 96, 97, 98; vaccinations 89, 96;
    when coping with uncertainty and risk
    generates further uncertainty and risk 92–3;
    witches 84, 91, 94
Mythen, G. 3, 63, 64, 65–6, 76, 80
myths 28, 120

Nagatake, T. 106
Namihira, E. 102

Naono, A. 96
Native Americans 28
natural disasters 120; threat of see risk society
    thesis: flood risk and poverty in Jakarta
Nazi Germany 67, 124
Neal, A. W. 43
neocolonialism 13
neoliberalism 6, 45
Norway: Sámi women 37–8
nuclear disasters 63, 66
Nuer-Dinka 30
Nugent, S. 65, 72

Obbo, C. 13
Obeyesekere, G. 80
Oedipus myths 28
Ohnuki-Tierney, E. 5, 102, 112, 114
Okada, S. 120
O'Keefe, P. 63
Olds, K. 45
Ong, A. 43, 45
oracles 29; Azande 25–6, 27, 37, 138
O'Reilly, K. 43
Ōta, T. 128
otherness 32, 74
Outhwaite, W. 2
outsiders 29, 32, 35, 64, 102, 112, 123, 137,
    138

pangolin 31, 33
paternalism 96
Philippi, D. 135
Piper, N. 43
pluralism, therapeutic 8, 93, 95, 96–8; health,
    risk and 79–81
political science 43
politics of risk 66–7; blaming the victim 73–5,
    76
Portes, A. 47
postcolonialism 4, 13
Pottier, R. 80, 93, 95
poverty see risk society thesis: flood risk and
    poverty in Jakarta
power relations 73–6
premodern Japan, control of danger in 5,
    118–40; doctors on Izu islands 123–4;
    findings 128–35; methodology 126–7;
    modern Japan 124–5; modernisation of Japan
    123–4, 139–40; plague demons
    (kegarawashiki eyami no oni) 120–1;
    premodern magical rituals in contemporary
    practices 131–5; risk, boundaries and
    pollution 119–20; shamanistic experts
    (Urabe) 120, 121, 122–3, 125, 127, 128,
    129–31, 132, 134, 135, 136, 138; trance
    states 122–3, 138, 139
psychosis 8
Pugh, J. F. 84

INDEX

Quinn, C. H. 69

Radcliffe-Brown, K. R. 126
rationality 3, 4–6, 8, 9; risk and 43–5; risk and mixed rationalities 56–8
religion 3, 7–8, 27, 119; fundamentalism 39; globalisation, magic and 36–9; hybrid forms of 39, 134; Indonesian labour migrants: faith and uncertainty 6, 42–58; Japan 120, 123, 132, 134, 136, 138, 140; Myanmar: Buddhism 6, 80, 82, 83, 85, 86, 87, 88, 89, 90, 92–3, 95, 97; typologies of societies: magic, science and 34–6
Renn, O. 44
Rice, G. 104
risk society thesis: flood risk and poverty in Jakarta 5, 62–76; abstract risk for actors in non-Western world 72–3; applicability of risk society theory outside late-modern society 62–7; changing nature of risk 63–4; class 62, 63, 64, 72, 73, 75–6; coping strategies 70, 71–2; discussion 75–6; findings 70–5; floods: old or new risk 70–1, 76; floods are (un)democratic 71–2; globalisation 62, 63, 65–6; informal settlement 71, 73–5; methodology 68–70; politics of risk: blaming the victim 73–5, 76; risk mapping 68–9; urbanisation 70–1
Rodlach, A. 15
Rome, ancient 22, 34–5
Rosa, E. A. 13
Rose, N. 102
Rosu, A. 94
Roth, J. A. 7, 38–9
Rothstein, H. 2
Rousseau, J.-J. 22
Russia 124

Sagala, S. 71
Saitō, H. 127, 134–5, 136
Satomura, K. 106
Schoepf, B. G. 13
science 3, 36, 37, 40, 119, 139; magic in modern systems 38–9; scientific paradigm: risk and health 13; typologies of societies: magic, religion and 34–6
Scotland 113
Scott, J. 64
Seale, C. 8
Seidel, G. 13
self-management 102
Setel, P. 13
shamans 128–34, 136, 137, 138, 139; Urabe 120, 121, 122–3, 125, 127, 128, 129–31, 132, 134, 135, 136, 138
Shilling, C. 8
Shim, J. 102, 113
Shintōism 123, 136, 138

Shiraishi, T. 106
Siahpush, M. 8
Siberia 94
Silvey, R. 43
Singapore: Indonesian labour migrants 42–58
Skidmore, M. 80, 96
Smith, D. J. 13
Smith, K. P. 13
social anthropology see anthropology
social order 32, 67, 74, 87, 119–20, 136
sociology 34, 43, 64
sorcery 4, 15, 29, 30, 33, 35, 37; Rakhine (Myanmar) 84
South Africa 15
Spanish flu pandemic (1918–1919) 104
Spinoza, B. 3, 6
spirits: Japan 125, 128, 129, 132, 135; Rakhine (Myanmar) 84, 87, 90–1
Spiro, M. E. 80, 94
SteelFisher, G. K. 104
structural functionalism 14
sub-Saharan Africa 4, 7, 12–13, 18; implications of methodologies for understanding risk 14, 16–17; intestinal worms (mchango) 17; linguistic relevance of risk in 14–16; misfortune 13–14, 15; risk in 13–14
subsistence farming 15
Suzuki, M. 102
Swearer, D. K. 80
Swidler, A. 13
syncretic or bricolaging approaches 3, 9
Szmukler, G. 8

taboos 32, 67, 95, 119
Tacitus 22
Takagi, K. 136
Tansey, J. 67
Tanzania 5, 12–18, 94, 95
Taoism 120
Tarrius, A. 48
Texier, P. 68, 70, 71
Thailand 94
therapeutic pluralism 8, 93, 95, 96–8; health, risk and 79–81
Torres Strait Islands 23, 36
tourism 37, 87, 124, 125, 127, 136
traditional healer 17, 89–90
Traphagan, J. W. 102, 114
Trobriand Islands 4, 23, 24–5, 33, 37, 39
Tsuchiya, H. 132
tuberculosis 7, 38–9
Tulloch, J. 16, 95, 97
Turner, B. S. 39

Umeno, M. 127, 136
United Kingdom 2, 65, 76, 80, 124; England 32, 35, 63; prevention of influenza: The Lancet 104; Scotland 113

INDEX

United States 3, 104, 106, 107, 108, 124
University of Cambridge 23

vaccinations 89, 96
Van Gennep, A. 32
Van Loon, J. 2
Van Voorst, R. 2, 3, 5, 6, 70, 72
Veltz, P. 45
Vertovec, S. 47

Wada, K. 103
Wallman, S. 13
Warner, J. 7, 8
Watt, A. 3
Weber, E. U. 65
Weber, M. 8
Weick, K. E. 49
Whyte, S. 13
Whyte, W.F. 27
Wilkinson, I. 2, 3, 66
Williams, A. M. 43

witchcraft 4, 7, 15, 29–30, 33, 34, 35–6; Azande
  26–7, 37, 40, 138, 139; Rakhine (Myanmar)
  84, 91, 94
women 67, 111, 114, 132; breast-feeding 8;
  Indonesian labour migrants 46, 47, 49; Japan:
  shamans (*Miko*) 122, 123, 127, 128, 132–4;
  Rakhine (Myanmar) 84, 86, 87, 88, 89, 94–5;
  Sámi women 37–8
Wong, D. 47
World Health Organization (WHO) 103

Yamada, H. 106
Yang, D. 43
Yasuhara, T. 106
Yeoh, B. S. A. 43
Yoro, T. 102
Young, M. W. 36, 37

Zelizer, V. 7
Zimbabwe 15
Zinn, J. 6, 8, 9, 18, 24, 25, 44, 47, 52, 57, 58

148